COLLABORATIVE HEALTH CARE

COLLABORATIVE HEALTH CARE

A Family-Oriented Model

Michael L. Glenn, M.D.

PRAEGER

New York
Westport, Connecticut
London

Library of Congress Cataloging-in-Publication Data

Glenn, Michael L. (Michael Lyon), 1938–
⌐ Collaborative health care.

  Bibliography: p.
  1. Family medicine. 2. Medical referral.
3. Holistic medicine. I. Title. [DNLM:
1. Community Medicine. 2. Family Practice.
W 84.5 G558c]
R729.5.G4G49 1987   616   87-2420
ISBN 0-275-92319-3 (alk. paper)

Library of Congress Catalog Card Number: 87-2420
ISBN: 0-275-92319-3

First published in 1987

Praeger Publishers, 521 Fifth Avenue, New York, NY 10175
A division of Greenwood Press, Inc.

Printed in the United States of America

∞

The paper used in this book complies with the Permanent
Paper Standard issued by the National Information Standards
Organization (Z39.48-1984).

10 9 8 7 6 5 4 3 2 1

CONTENTS

Preface   *vii*

Acknowledgments   *xv*

PART I

Chapter

1   The Context of Health Care Today   3

2   What's Already Known   16

3   Some Basic Notions   35

4   What's Already Been Tried: Antecedents   57

5   What's Been Tried: 1945 to the Present   69

6   The Organization of Collaborative Health Care   88

PART II

7   Collaborative Health Care in Practice   105

8   Starting Up   130

9   A Sampler: Clinical Examples of
     Collaborative Health Care   138

10   Problems in Collaboration   160

11   Referral to the Therapist   180

12   Questions Frequently Asked about CHC   195

13   Summary   203

Bibliography   *205*

Index   *213*

About the Author   *221*

PREFACE

The basic outlines of what has come to be called "family systems medicine" have now been laid forth. This contextual approach to medical care emphasizes the interrelationship of psychosocial and bio-medical factors in illness and its treatment. It focuses on ways in which the family unit both affects and is affected by sickness in any of its members. The use of systems thinking sharpens a view of illness as an evolving process: illness is seen as a patterned phenomenon rather than an isolated time-bound thing, as a socially defined entity rather than a simple physiological event, as a dynamic process rather than as straightforward cause and effect. The core theories of this approach, its perspective, and its contextual insistence have already been described. The studies that validate these concepts and ideas have been accumulating for the past 30 years; and, while they may still seem new in some circles, their overall coherence and strength is already a fait accompli.

Yet, in all of this, something has gone wrong: The organization of health care which should reflect such a systemic world view has not developed, and in fact lags far behind the advances in theory. A broader view of health and illness suggests that health care should be an interdisciplinary process, uniting the efforts and skills of different health professionals. Responding to social, political, cultural, and economic conditions, however, the organization of health care services is now marked by a paradoxical resurgence of the biomedical model: specialist care, fragmentation of services—a world view that seemed passe 20 years ago, supposedly superceded in medicine by the bio-psychosocial model of health and illness.

A long-range view suggests that this is not surprising. The transformation of ideas into practice is a difficult process and it often lingers behind the development of the ideas themselves; deep resistance frequently opposes any kind of change. An integrated health care system may yet develop, although it is not a given by any means. The current trends that oppose such care require careful investigation and analysis. Are they simply part of the dialectical process of inevitable change, or do they instead signal the decline of the biopsychosocial model as a force which affects the actual delivery of health care?

Given the increased enthusiasm in some quarters for an integrated approach, we need to examine what forms of organization family systems medicine adherents could pursue in practice. Several attempts of this type have already been tried, and many collaborative practices now exist. This book advocates a model of health care that, in its general outlines, is both collaborative and family-oriented. Closely following the principles of family systems medicine, it is offered as a guide to giving better health care to the public.

COLLABORATIVE HEALTH CARE

What is collaborative health care? Simply put, it is health care provided by several health professionals who work closely together, trying to offer more comprehensive care than usually is available. Care, for example, may be given to aspects of preventive medicine and to the psychosocial ills afflicting patients and their families. Which health professionals are involved? How closely together do they work? These questions are more complicated.

Often (but not always) the family (or primary care) physician is the patient or family's main health care provider, offering more comprehensive treatment through his or her association with counseling or therapy professionals, a social worker, or someone else who can deal with patients' psychological and/or social needs. This can take place in the private as well as the public sector; in fee-for-service, HMO (prepaid), clinic, or institutional settings. It can occur in a solo practice or in a group medical practice. The counselor may be on salary, receive a percentage of what s/he brings in, or work on a fee-for-service basis. Collaboration may occur entirely within a single practice or in a single location, such as a medical office building, where several physicians work closely with a therapist through referrals and follow-up. It may even occur when a physician refers to certain counselors across town and then follows up and coordinates care with these counselors.

Collaborative health care is not new. Several of its forms have a long tradition, such as the interdisciplinary arrangements found in large hospitals, training and teaching settings, and some clinics and community health centers. Other forms have developed relatively recently, such as counselors working in private physicians' offices or the comprehensive care offered by a health maintenance organization (HMO). The roots of collaborative health care go back to the traditions of social medicine, to collaborative public health programs in the late nineteenth century, and to medical social work, which dates back to the early 1900s. Notable collaborative projects in this century include the Peckham Experiment in Great Britain in the 1930s and the Macy Foundation project in the 1940s. The latter explored providing comprehensive family-based care in New York and led to the book *Patients Have Families* by H. B. Richardson (1948). The 1960s saw dozens of attempts to bring a collaborative team approach to community health issues. These efforts involved hundreds of physicians, nurses, community-based professionals and paraprofessionals, social workers, physician extenders, therapists, and patients themselves. Rather than constituting a new development, efforts to work collaboratively around health care issues should be viewed as a constant historical trend: rising, falling, now rising again.

The trend has some characteristic features. It places health care in a context that transcends the biomedical model. It argues that health care must treat the "whole person," not just organ systems, and holds that such care is often best provided in a family or social context. It tries to emphasize health as much as disease, to look into preventive medicine as much as to crisis care, and to avoid the language of pathophysiology (dysfunction) and pathological anatomy (diseased organs). In addition, it understands that providing health care demands more than one health care provider and more than one health care discipline or profession; it leans towards health care teams or integrated practice rather than toward the primacy of any one health care profession. Finally, it holds that providers themselves are part of the health care process, not wholly detached and dispassionate scientific observers.

After a decade of relative decline, interdisciplinary work in health care is resurfacing today. Unlike previous efforts, this resurgence depends on the simultaneous growth of two new fields: family medicine and family therapy. Family medicine did not exist 20 years ago, and family therapy was still defining itself then. Today, both fields are successful, and practitioners in each are increasingly interested in the organic and behavioral problems that accompany physical illness. Family therapy has influenced the growth of other mental health fields, too, such as marriage and family, and social work counseling. As Doherty and Baird have noted (1983), family therapy and family medicine are "natural allies." Each looks at the context in which illness occurs. Each is especially concerned with the dynamics of the family. The core personnel for developing collaborative health care today can thus be found among these family physicians and family therapists. They join the other health professionals—nurses, social workers, and other primary care physicians—who have been working together in the area of health and the family for decades.

The core notion behind collaborative health care (CHC) is to join a concern with the traditional biomedical dimensions of health care with an attention to psychosocial (especially family) factors affecting health and sickness. Typically, the physicians will handle their patients' physical complaints, but they will also inquire as to concurrent emotional stresses. They may engage in brief counseling themselves, and/or they may refer patients who need further counseling to their colleagues for mental health, educative or psychotherapy services. Counseling will also be undertaken around issues such as noncompliance with medical treatment, family conflicts (life-stage and life-cycle issues, issues involving more than one member of the family), and symptoms that appear to be psychosomatic, that is, which apparently involve psychological as well as biomedical factors in their development and presentation.

Collaborative practices may function as "gatekeepers" of medical care, treating whatever problems they can, and referring patients for more specialized treatment when necessary. Hospitalization would be carried out, when appropriate, in an affiliated community or tertiary-care facility. Care provided this way can prove cost-effective, satisfying to patients, and in the interests of the public's health in the long run.

Guided by this general orientation, many practitioners are currently developing their own version of collaborative care. The field is so new that nobody can dogmatically define it now. Nobody can say what collaborative care "has to" look like. A variety of experiences is being forged. We thus need to gather and share people's experiences, sift through what is known, and begin developing shared guidelines for such activity.

In spite of the enthusiasm that has been generated, collaborative health care is far from a swelling trend. In fact, it is struggling for its life. Economic and political trends reward the fragmentation of health care provided along the lines of the old model: specialties and sub-specialties; procedures, tests, and operations. Yet a collaborative alternative makes sense for everyone involved; physicians, patients and their families, as well as for those who provide the final health care dollar. It can keep medical costs down as well as (if not better than) any other model, while at the same time offering the accessibility and continuity of care that patients want. It is care that comprehends an individual patient's distress by situating him or her in a broader context, and thus corresponds better to our cor.temporary understanding of health and illness than do models built around the old biomedical view.

This book appears as more and more health professionals—physicians, nurses, therapists, social workers, counselors, educators—are in fact working together to provide comprehensive health care for their patients. Although these professionals work in different settings and are reimbursed in different ways, they are united by a conviction that health care requires a multidisciplinary approach, because providers cannot provide comprehensive health care on their own.

A conviction in itself, however, will not create a groundswell for collaborative care. Only concrete incentives to such care can do that. The main questions are: Can providers be reimbursed for what they do? Will the large health care organizations adopt a long-term or a short-term view of their tasks, a view encouraging fragmented, biomedically oriented care or one promoting comprehensive, prevention-oriented care? The answers to these questions are not clear, but they will affect the future of the model this book describes.

INTERDISCIPLINARY PERSPECTIVE

Some books and articles have touched on aspects of collaborative care, but most view it from only one field's perspective. To advance our understanding, we need a shared interdisciplinary perspective, reaching out to practitioners of many persuasions. The appearance of the periodical *Family Systems Medicine* represents one effort to create an interdisciplinary, archival journal in the field. A kindred effort is the development of the (regrettably short-lived) user newsletter "Working Together." Similar efforts include the historical development of multidisciplinary departments of family medicine, the experiences with community health care teams in the late 1960s and early 1970s, and current work around community-oriented primary care in groups such as the American Public Health Association.

Without an interdisciplinary perspective, practitioners from different fields are left within the strictures of their own professional training. Problems that arise early on in the course of trying to develop a collaborative practice will seem to stem from personality differences or from not trying hard enough, instead of from the particular differences in outlook and philosophy that people from different fields bring with them. The first step in breaking down such differences is to recognize and respect the history and accomplishment of each collegial field, and to sift out differences by charting each discipline's hierarchies, assumed beliefs, language, and basic goals. I hope that this volume can help collaborators understand each other better.

Still missing from most of the published discussion on collaborative health care work are voices of the on-line professionals (not academics) who are already working collaboratively to provide hands-on care to patients and clients. Many of these professionals are working in isolation from one another, unaware that others are doing similar things. Often, professionals only know material about the collaborative process that's been written from their own particular discipline, and are unaware of material from other disciplines.

This book is addressed both to those practitioners who are interested in working in a collaborative health care setting and to health policy planners who are concerned with developing health care systems that improve the current organization and delivery of health care. It should also be of interest to a variety of health professionals in training programs who are considering the direction of their careers.

The book is divided into two main parts. Part I presents an analysis of the trends germane to the development of collaborative health care. It provides a thematic and historical overview. My sense is that even many people committed to collaborative health care do not know the history and traditions of their own efforts. Those interested in this sort of analytical overview will find basic background material here. Part II is a more practical description of collaborative health care practice as it currently exists. Here, I describe the guidelines of such practice, variants of the model, and offer case examples of actual collaborative work. People interested more in this pragmatic aspect of the topic will find Part II more applicable to their concerns.

Throughout, I have tried to present the material in a direct way, so that interested readers will not have to struggle their way through the diverse jargons that each health care profession has managed to accrue. Indeed, one of the greatest obstacles to any working together is having to translate from the language and perspective of one field to the language and very different perspective of the others.

A PERSONAL NOTE

My ideas are not divorced from my own career. I originally entered medicine with the idea of becoming a family physician. In medical school in the early 1960s, I became more and more attracted to psychiatry, and to the areas of overlap between psychodynamics and physical illness. One of the first projects I ever worked on was with

Dr. Donald Kornfeld at Columbia College of Physicians & Surgeons, looking into the subjective experiences of people who had survived a heart attack. Later in medical school I obtained permission to follow a handful of patients with serious, chronic illnesses—a girl with Hand-Schuller-Christian disease, an adolescent with cystic fibrosis. After taking a "mixed medical" internship, which covered neurology, pediatrics, and internal medicine, I entered psychiatric residency.

My experience was mixed. The New York State Psychiatric Institute's orientation then was heavily "individual," whereas I was drawn instead to the more dramatic fields of group and family therapy, which my teachers tended to scorn. Thanks to a remarkable elective with Nat Ackerman (at the Family Institute in New York City, which now bears his name), however, I was fortunate enough to find fertile soil for my ideas, as well as the friendship and support of therapists such as Don Bloch, Phoebe Prosky, Kitty LaPerriere, and Judith Lieb.

In the 1960s I became active in more political aspects of therapy. I began *The Radical Therapist*, worked in alternative settings as well as with family therapists—especially David Kantor—and then eventually left therapy entirely. When I reentered medical practice, it was as a family physician. I felt I could make a better contribution to people's overall health as a family doctor than as a psychiatrist.

As I learned more about family medicine, I came to appreciate its unique position among the medical specialties. Only family medicine had a genuinely broad perspective. It was the only field whose faculty was so interdisciplinary, so influenced by the social sciences. I gradually met leaders in the field, and began to analyze the ideological struggles that were taking place in it.

In my own practice, I knew I was unable to provide both the medical and the counseling help that was needed. A turning point came when I attended a conference at Skidmore in 1981 on "Family Therapy and Family Medicine." The speakers included Jack Medalie, Macaran Baird, and Janet Christie-Seely. I went with Barry Dym, a family therapist whom I'd met through Dave Kantor. Barry and I had already been talking about collaboration between therapists and physicians, and he had just started the Boston Center for Family Health, whose therapist staff was interested in working with the problems that arose in families with a physically ill member. The Skidmore meeting galvanized us into thinking further about how family medicine and family therapy could work together around problems encountered in primary medical care.

The meeting spurred me to bring a family therapist into my own family practice to help out with the psychosocial aspects of my patients' problems. At Skidmore I met Martin Cohen, Elizabeth Keating-Cohen, and Linda Atkins, all of whom have now worked as therapists at our Everett Family Practice. I preferred to limit my own treatment role to recognizing such problems, not carrying out psychotherapy. I adopted the kind of work Janet Christie-Seely calls "working with the family"—working with my patients from an understanding of their family and social context, but not initiating family therapy, per se.

It was also at the Skidmore conference that Barry and I met with Don Bloch and agreed to begin the journal *Family Systems Medicine*. That was an exciting time, indeed—the source of much later work and many friendships.

The idea of collaborative care has thus been developing for some time. Its actual crystallization came in a walk with Don Bloch, who suggested that the large number of marriage and family counselors was the therapist component which could be allied with family physicians to provide basic medical care. Barry came up with the term *primary care therapist*, as did Mac Baird and Bill Doherty at about the same time. (Very few ideas in this book are uniquely my own.) Over the last few years, though, I've felt it increasingly important to write an advocate position for this model of medical care. I've watched family medicine edge away from its contextual view of care, and I've watched comprehensive medical services become less and less available to people in my own community. The resurgence of the biomedical model seems a cruel mockery of all that had been learned about the psychosocial dimensions of medical care over the past 30 years, and it seems due to mainly economic factors and Reaganomics.

So it was that I determined to write a history of collaborative care and present its case to those who would listen.

ACKNOWLEDGMENTS

My style is my own, but I can't say the same about my ideas. I owe much to others. Donald Kornfeld first inspired me to consider this broad area of care. Nat Ackerman, David Kantor, Kitty Laperriere, and Phoebe Prosky helped whet my interest in family dynamics. Don Bloch and Barry Dym have been indefatigable, inspirational colleagues. So have a number of friends in family medicine—Don Ransom most especially, whose keen mind has led family medicine for years; G. Gayle Stephens, whose bold views, panoramic perspective, and deep moral sense, as well as his capacity for new visions continues to astound and inspire me; Lucy Candib, an early friend and dedicated thinker in the field; Janet Christie-Seely, Mac Baird, Jack Medalie, Don Cassata, Shae Kosch, and others on the STFM Task Force on the Family in Family Medicine. My colleague Robert Singer has been a help in formulating many of my ideas, and his being in the practice has given me the time to write. Therapists Linda Atkins and Martin Cohen have contributed to my ideas, especially through our case discussions. Rita Ulrich has been a source of much energy, in reflecting on her own collaborative experience in the Valentine Lane project. Others have also been helpful over the years: Janet Bunbury who is connected with the Peckham Experiment, Larry Mauksch and William Phillips whose interview was very stimulating to me, Ron and Binnie Backer who work as a husband/wife physician/therapist team in nearby Winchester. To all these people and others, I am most grateful.

PART ONE

ONE

The Context of
Health Care Today

Collaborative health care must be understood in the context of health care today, when the organization of health care services is changing more rapidly than ever before. Starr (1983) has described the transformation of U.S. medicine from a concern of small-time doctor-entrepreneurs and/or local hospitals into a huge business run mainly for profit and increasingly dominated by nationwide corporate giants. The solo practitioner is becoming a vanishing species. Even private practice itself is under siege, as greater and greater numbers of HMOs and other prepaid programs attempt to lock in the employed (therefore better situated) consumers of medical care. The large health care chains, able to depend on substantial amounts of capital, hire physicians and other professionals to provide whatever health care services their managers think are profitable for them to offer. The number of private group practices and PPOs (physicians in private practice who form an HMO-type group) are both growing, but the economics of medical care are increasingly pushing physicians to work for larger health care organizations.

Society's concept of health care is constantly being redefined. Whereas 20 years ago the prevailing trend was toward broadening the notion of health care and making services accessible to all strata of the population, now the trend is towards conceiving such services more narrowly and limiting them, thus denying many people access to care on economic grounds. Whereas 25 years ago health care was enthusiastically being asked to cope with a broad variety of ills affecting

3

people's health—bringing in occupational, nutritional, environmental, and psychological issues—now the pendulum has swung to the idea that less is better, and that certain kinds of care should not be included under everyone's umbrella. Although, 25 years ago, notions of health care had expanded to include preventive medicine, maternal and child care, as well as a new focus on community and family health, trends now are to move away from such issues as not "cost-effective." Earlier, people talked about the shortage of physicians in primary care fields; now, although this shortage still exists (!), we hear more about the "doctor glut," and programs affecting family and community health—immunizations, school breakfasts and lunches, WIC (Women and Infant Care), food stamps, community health centers—are being trimmed from federal and state budgets.

Physicians and others concerned with health have spoken out over the past three decades about helping patients cope with the psychosocial stresses that engender and abet physical illness. The move today is away from this position. Following the criticisms of Ivan Illich (1976) and some health care consumers, the fashionable argument now is that life has been "over-medicalized." By this, it is implied either that too many social problems or problems in daily life have been described as illnesses, and thus handed over to the medical establishment for treatment, or else that physicians have been given too much power for decisions in general. Thomas Szasz (1974) has criticized the tendency to label "deviant" behavior—people's ways of life—as diseases. The overall implication of this critique is that medical care is bad for your health. Think of all the iatrogenic diseases, adverse effects of medications, unnecessary surgery, physicians' errors in diagnosis and treatment. The conclusion is that physicians, therapists and other health care professionals should pull back. How ironic that the libertarian critique dovetails with the conservative attempt to limit medical services so as to cut medical costs.

These developments have critically affected the movement for more accessible health care, a movement which last surged in the 1960s. It then threatened to topple the dominant biomedical model of health and disease and supplant it with a wider "biopsychosocial" view. Accompanying this assault at an ideological level were attempts in the late 1960s and early 1970s actually to change the way health care was delivered. Prominent in such efforts were projects to provide care via interdisciplinary teams and to develop a community base for health care services. Now these efforts have ended, and the pendulum is swinging in the other direction.

Earlier 1950s notions of health and disease are being restored, while at the same time the patient-practitioner relationship is being undermined. The current corporatization of health care treats health care like any other commodity: an item for sale, whose delivery should turn a profit. Amidst this transformation, the sancrosanct doctor-patient relationship is being redefined in terms of its cost-effectiveness. Fiscal intermediaries now determine the parameters of care. At a time when individual physicians are being sued in record numbers for malpractice (and for record amounts), the power of individual doctors actually to control their patients' care has markedly diminished. Physicians must follow the new corporate or federal cost-control rules—or else. Their much-touted autonomy is being eroded. As for the "biopsychosocial" model, current incentives encourage medical care once again to be fragmented among provider professionals, even as it is being concentrated among providing organizations. Diagnostic (and, therefore, reimbursement) codes continue to follow organ-system, not whole-person, medical problems, and the insurance industry continues to decide diagnostic nosology. New rules guiding access to care mean that individual physicians, whether in- or outside of HMOs, often cannot provide what their patients want—hospitalization, referral to a specialist, diagnostic procedures. At the same time preventive services and other services aimed at the psychosocial dimensions of health care have increasingly become nonreimbursable. (Who will provide it free?) A side phenomenon of all this is the recasting of psychiatric thought into biomedical molds: psychiatrists are now relabeling many illnesses as essentially genetic or biochemical diseases. If they don't treat a disorder with tricyclic antidepressants, they treat it with Lithium. "Talking therapy" is not only less reimbursable, it is falling out of favor with the *cognoscenti*.

Of course, while doing this, few health care planners bother to ask the public what it wants. The question, "How can the health needs of patients and their families best be served?" is not on their docket. Nor has effort gone into examining what forms of health care organization can encourage health promotion, prevent disease, and/or ease the burden of illness on patients and their loved ones.

In the past three decades, we have learned an amazing amount about the interrelationships between stress factors, family dynamics, and physical illness. Yet I'm afraid that much of this knowledge is being abandoned, mainly because of economic considerations, and partly because people are not yet convinced of its importance. My thesis is that some collaborative form of health care is best suited to people's needs and wants. It is a model based on close work between family, primary care physicians and family-oriented health-care counselors; and it can be practiced in almost any kind of health care setting. Such care rests on the view that health care is multidimensional, and the recognition that people prefer receiving health care in a family- or community-oriented way.

To understand the potential of this collaborative model built around the primary care physician, let me first review the history of family practice in the United States.

THE FAMILY PHYSICIAN

Many studies show that Americans, given a choice, prefer having a family doctor who cares for the daily medical woes of the whole family. They want a constant and accessible physician who has known them over the years. This is true in spite of the rhetoric of specialist medical care, which implies that specialist medicine is the only "good" medicine, and that people should no longer seek out health care generalists who treat patients as whole people in a family context.

Years ago, most physicians were generalists: in 1932, 85 percent of U.S. physicians were general practitioners. The development of specialist medical care after World War II changed that. A tremendous acceleration of medical technology occurred between 1945 and 1955, and by 1970 the prewar situation had been completely reversed: 85 percent of physicians were specialists, and general practice was virtually dead. The rise of medical specialization meant that most Americans no longer had the family doctor they wanted.

The image of a humanistic, compassionate family physician seems almost anachronistic; and yet, in recent years, the family doctor has made a dramatic comeback. Begun in 1969, family medicine has become the fastest growing medical specialty in the United States, with over 400 residency programs and about 15 percent of current medical school graduates.

Family practice is not just "another" primary care specialty. Its birth in the 1960s was the product of a reformist movement attempting to restore a humanistic approach to medical care. Advocating the care of the "whole person" in his or her family context, it opposed the growing fragmentation of modern medical care. Many of family medicine's early leaders were practicing physicians. They were attracted to the new discipline because it embraced the many factors they knew were important in family health care, psychosocial as well as biomedical. Today, the orientation of family practice still contrasts with the rest of organized medicine, where specialists busily refer to one another, each taking care of a different member of the family and a different organ system.

What was said above about the tenor of family medicine holds equally true, however, for many physicians in other primary care fields, such as internal medicine and pediatrics. Throughout the medical system, one finds practitioners whose work emanates from their understanding that disease involves more than pathogens and that health involves many mixed physical and psychological factors. These physicians' practices are informed by their grasp of the psychosocial dimensions of medical phenomena.

THE PSYCHOSOCIAL DIMENSIONS OF CARE

It's long been known that patients present their physician with significant psychosocial problems and concerns. The President's Commission on Mental Health (Report to the President, 1978) recognized this, stating that "far greater numbers of people with emotional problems turn to primary health care providers than to mental health practitioners when they first seek help." Studies from our practice in Everett (Glenn et al., 1984) show that between 10 and 20 percent of all patients' visits are characterized by a significant psychosocial problem, strong enough for psychotherapy to be considered as a treatment modality. These figures agree with earlier data from the Health Care Center Plan of Greater New Haven (Coleman, 1983) showing that "about 15 percent of the patients presented psychiatric complaints to their physicians during a two-year study period. About 70 percent of these psychiatric problems were looked after by primary clinicians on their own" (p. 113).

Attention to the psychosocial dimensions of patients' problems is generally acknowledged as being one of the main and unique features of family practice (Medalie, 1978; Rakel, 1983; Taylor, 1983), yet estimates of the overall frequency of such problems vary widely within the field, from 3 percent (Rosenblatt et al., 1982) to 80 percent (Carmichael and Carmichael, 1981), thus reflecting a wide gamut of opinion on the subject. The variation shows divergent views on the relevance of patients' psychosocial problems to their medical care. On one end stand practitioners with a principally biomedical orientation. Although they may acknowledge that their patients' complaints are situated in a matrix of psychosocial factors, they mainly focus on the medical reasons for the visit. For example, Rosenblatt et al.'s study on the content of family practice (1982) attributes a frequency of only 3 percent to the diagnostic cluster of "anxiety/depression," its *sole* psychosocial diagnostic category.

A midrange position is reflected in a previous paper from our practice (1984), which notes that between 10 and 20 percent of patients seen over a 12-month period were judged likely to benefit from psychotherapeutic intervention. The group included people with major symptoms of anxiety, depression, and acute situational stress reactions; psychotic behavior; stress-related illnesses such as tension headaches, irritible bowel syndrome, neurodermatitis; and hypochondriasis or "somatic fixation" (Huygen and Smits, 1983) upon various organ systems.

A more ambitious view could easily argue that 60 to 100 percent of patient visits involve important psychosocial issues. This position comes from those who describe the "relational" aspect of family practice as one of its basic features (Carmichael and Carmichael, 1981) as well as from those who affirm that, since psychosocial issues are present in *every* human encounter, they are present in medical encounters, too, and physicians should deal with them more often (Dym, 1984). Many patients are worried by such issues, they point out, but do not raise them spontaneously; instead, they wait for their physician to ask. Recognizing this, and holding to the doctor-patient relationship as the keystone of family practice, Carmichael and Carmichael (1981) have estimated that the "relational model" of family practice, which mainly focuses on providing care and comfort over time, and which deals with the continuing broad range of issues affecting patients' lives, comprises approximately 80 percent of clinical family practice. They feel many fewer encounters focus around making a biomedical diagnosis (the "clinical model") or dealing with forms, certificates, and so on (the "adversarial model"). This view is akin to Balint's (1957) and to the views of other humanizers of medical care, especially Stephens (1982).

Each position on the spectrum argues with those on either side of it. At stake however is the future of medical care: towards greater or lesser involvement with the "whole" picture, a wider or a more restricted view of health care.

Today's family-oriented physicians hold that the family (or household) is a basic unit of health care; they also look into other ecological health care factors—workplace, school, and community. These physicians view health and illness in a systemic way, following the "continuum" and "hierarchy" of natural and social systems (Engel, 1977). They attempt more education and preventive medicine, and are concerned with promoting health, not just treating disease.

FAMILY THERAPY

Family therapy has also grown enormously over the past decades since its modest beginnings in the 1950s. Having reached a more mature stage, some of its practitioners have now begun to examine psychodynamic and other therapy-related questions surrounding physical illness. Recent trends in this field have included looking into the family context of patients suffering from a wide variety of medical problems and trying to describe the patterns of behavior occurring around acute illness, chronic illness, disability, and so on. Family therapists have become involved in hospice care, pastoral counseling, marital therapy, grief work, and substance abuse, to name only a few areas of potential overlap with primary care physicians.

Now more and more therapists and counselors are seeing the advantages of collaborating with physicians, especially since it gives them access to patients who can use their special skills—an understanding of communication, the ability to understand family dynamics, an acceptance of a systemic perspective—and whom they would otherwise not treat. They want to become even more involved with areas of family health, and with the physical and emotional problems that arise in the course of family life.

Primary care (family) physicians, practicing collaboratively with primary care (family) therapists, can together care for the vast majority of people's everyday medical and psychological problems—and in an integrated fashion. There will be far less temptation to foster the so-called "mind/body split" and more opportunity to practice holistic, comprehensive care. To do this will require serious changes in the model and organization of medical care.

QUESTIONS OF COST

Medicine today has become a vast money-making enterprise (Ginzberg, 1984). Profits can be made, mainly by fitting treatment into the traditional diagnostic categories. Relying upon diagnostic codes that are wedded to the biomedical model of disease, the insurance industry today dictates payment for medical services and structures the way these services are conceptualized. Almost all incentives to make money through the provision of health care have been locked into the old ways of thinking about medical problems.

Concern with escalating health care costs has been the main propelling agent so far to health care reorganization. Worry over the cost of medical care is indeed appropriate. Medical care expenses have steadily increased in the past 40 years. The cost of medical care expenditures has mushroomed from $22 billion in 1960, to $60 billion in 1970, and to $287 billion in 1981, 9.8 percent of the gross national product (GNP). The estimate was for an expenditure of $438 billion in 1985 (10.5% of GNP), $758 billion in 1990 (11.5% of GNP), and $1000 billion in the year 2000, unless some action is taken to halt the trend. Since Medicaid and Medicare were enacted in 1966, the government has assumed an ever-increasing percentage of total health-care costs (28% in 1979 as opposed to 13% in 1966 from the federal government, with another 12% from state and local governments). In addition, private health insurance paid 27 percent of the total medical care costs in 1979, leaving direct payment for services in 1979 at a historical low of 32 percent.

The new concern over costs has coincided with a shift in medical ethics and medical values. If physicians had become small-time businessmen, at least they had their other side, their concern for their patients and their willingness to stand advocate to their patients' needs. Corporations, however, have no such other side. They make no pretense to be anything but businesses. The corporations' assault on the health care consumer has meant the further commercialization of medical care, making it a commodity for promotion and for sale.

A number of economic factors are at work here:

• Medical care has become a potentially vast money-making enterprise (Ginsberg, 1984). More people have insurance coverage than ever before. There are profits to be made if one follows the rules and knows how to bill.

• More money goes to the people performing technological services, procedures, and operations than to those who care for patients in their office, treat chronic problems, talk to their patients, and so on.

• The insurance industry dictates payment for medical services. It does so through the use of diagnostic codes that are totally wedded to the biomedical model of disease. Thus, the financial incentives are locked to the "old ways" of thinking about medical problems.

• The emergence of larger and larger HMOs and of "corporate medicine"—large chains of hundreds of hospitals, nursing homes, emergency room facilities, and so on—has established the profit motive as the be-all and end-all in medical treatment. These developments can undercut the humanistic traditions of medicine, especially the importance of the doctor-patient relationship, and they may well retard the move toward a broader view of illness and disease. And yet, the particular structure of an HMO can actually encourage the development of collaborative forms of practice faster than might the strictly private sector.

THE RENAISSANCE OF THE BIOMEDICAL MODEL

One consequence of the concern with the ever-escalating costs of medical care has been a renaissance of the biomedical model of disease. Corporate medicine understands that reimbursement follows diagnosis, and today's diagnostic codes chop people up, organ system by organ system. The health care provider is reimbursed for procedures aimed at specific illnesses, and health care problems that do not easily fit into the standard diagnostic scheme wind up being nonreimbursable.

The triumph of specialist medicine in the post-World War II period has meant higher medical costs. Family practice and the other primary care specialties offer less costly care. Yet prepaid plans have until recently not promoted greater reliance on ambulatory care. For example, insurance programs have frequently covered care in emergency rooms (which by definition is an "emergency"), but not care in physicians' offices. In addition, many insurance plans fail to cover counseling services, even though studies show that preventive care, including attention to both medical and psychological problems, saves money and decreases distress in the long run. The current system is set up for urgent, critical care, not preventive care. Today's financial problems could well prompt a reexamination of this attitude, and try to reward medical programs that can decrease the overall number of hospital days, treat people in offices instead of emergency rooms, and develop ambulatory care. Until recently, however, it has been doing just the opposite.

The renaissance of the biomedical model is an ironic development, for it occurs just when the family systems approach was developing new insights into the experience of illness. Admitting a diversity of psychosocial factors to our notions of health and disease, the latter embraced a patient's family and/or community as the context in which illness and its treatment occurs, and thus helped deepen our understanding of the meaning and significance of any given disease.

Family-oriented counselors and therapists were working in hospitals, community health clinics, and with private physicians, applying their insights to problems associated with medical illness. The public seemed responsive to the notion of whole-person and "holistic" health care. Yet recent trends toward the corporatization of health care threaten to leave these new insights on the shelf. The corporate health planners have frequently accepted the old-fashioned model, because it is neater, and because it excludes much that they would just as soon keep excluded.

THE RISE OF THE HMOS:

Encouragement of the Family Practice Model?

The emergence of HMOs and corporate medicine—large chains of hospitals, nursing homes, emergency facilities, and so on—marks a new era in the organization of medical care. It threatens to undercut older humanistic traditions of medicine, including the sanctity of the doctor-patient relationship. Yet, if HMOs have a potential for cutting back on the broader view of illness and disease, they also have the material, economic basis for abandoning the biomedical model and its fragmented organization of care. HMOs pursuing a contextual, family approach could make the biopsychosocial model a reality. By following a collaborative model, they could decrease their health care costs in the long run, and thus pave the way for more accessible, less costly comprehensive care.

A number of new HMOs have seen this possibility, and they have begun to base all medical care around a family physician. This saves money by reducing unnecessary referrals to specialists and by reducing tests and expensive procedures. It also makes for more satisfied health care consumers, for the primary care (family) physician can offer continuous, more personal care. Family practice-oriented HMOs provide a challenge to the other HMOs, especially as most HMOs have shown little regard for the psychosocial areas affecting people's health: cutting mental health services from their program and focusing exclusively on physical illnesses in basically healthy people.

Not only will such an approach satisfy the consumer's wishes, but it can also cut health care costs. Studies from the Kaiser Permanente

HMO (Cummings and Follete, 1968; Follette and Cummings, 1967; Cummings, 1977) document a decrease in medical care costs when psychological counseling was offered as part of the plan, and an even further decrease when such care was offered without limits. This suggests that integrating counseling services into its program makes fiscal sense for the HMO as well as providing more complete health care for the consumer. The basic premise is, that attention to the psychosocial aspects of people's health, especially when undertaken early in the game, can help prevent the outbreak and exacerbation of disease processes, and can therefore save money in the long run.

Relying on family physicians as gatekeepers may also help control costs by emphasizing office- rather than hospital-based treatment.

The Model Described

Collaborative health care need not be the only form of health care organization. But it should be at least one of the models available in our pluralistic system. My sense is that, if it is available, it will prove both popular and cost-effective, and can become the basic model for health care services. Right now, however, the main challenge is just giving this model a chance.

Collaborative health care makes interdisciplinary health care teams the basic providers of primary health care. Its main personnel are family (or primary care) physicians and family therapists or counselors. Allied health personnel can be added as needed. Such groups can be organized into fairly small, easily duplicable community-based practices. Between three and seven providers overall is enough. This could exist under a private practice model. It could be in government-funded clinics. It could be organized in an HMO around small modular satellite clinics, each situated in a particular community and offering a more local, personal form of primary medical care.

The teams can also function as gatekeepers of care. They can refer patients to specialists and hospitalize patients in community hospitals as needed. Patients would have access to tertiary hospital care, too, if necessary. The concept of physicians as gatekeepers has gained some support in medical-economic circles. Physicians receive only 19 percent of the consumer's health care dollar, but they control much of how the remainder is spent through ordering tests, prescribing drugs, and hospitalizing patients. Hospital costs account for 41 percent of medical expenses. Drugs and appliances represent another 10 percent. If physicians could hold down costs—through decreasing unnecessary hospitalizations and unnecessary surgery, cutting down hospital stays, prescribing less costly drugs, and so on—the total cost of care would drop.

Care provided in such a continuous, available way by teams of family therapists and family physicians would prove (1) cost-effective, (2) satisfying to patients, (3) an avenue for further understanding and research in matters of health and disease. Following a biopsychosocial model, it would be both community-based and family-oriented. It would integrate approaches of trained family therapists and family physicians. It would deemphasize procedure-oriented medical care while reemphasizing continuous contact between family members and primary health care people—therapists, physicians, and others— who would follow family members through the decades of their lives, attending to their medical and psychological needs. A good model of this already in practice can be seen in Huygen's *Family Medicine* (1978).

THE REORGANIZATION OF HEALTH CARE

Currents in medical care today promise to transform it from something like a cottage industry linked up to local hospitals into the preserve of giant corporations. These currents begin with the monetarization of health care and the appropriation of health care resources by large corporations. Whatever else it is, medical care is also a commodity. A predominant motive for change, however, is to decrease overall health care costs while managing to provide a profit for the medical provider. The press toward for-profit hospitals, large specialist-based HMOs, PPOs, emergency centers, nursing home chains, and so on, can act to fragment medical care even further, limiting the understanding of illness narrowly to biomedicine; or it can encourage a more efficient, comprehensive approach to health care. A collaborative model is just as appropriate to an HMO with satellite community centers as it is to fee-for-profit private practice.

The rational reorganization of health care has several components. First, there are many *economic* and *political* aspects: the cost of medical care as now organized is simply too much for the country to support. Second, there are *personal* considerations: people in this country want a personal physician who will be available to them, and who will see them and their family over time and for a variety of physical, emotional, and other complaints. Third, there are *professional* considerations: what will become of the "calling" of medicine, its responsibility, its duty, its humanism. Fourth and last, there are theoretical and ideo-logical questions: which paradigm of illness will medical care pursue? Will it fall back to the biomedical model, which creates a disease for every encounter, or will it move towards a more holistic view of ill-ness, which includes familial and social factors, and which seeks to understand the meaning of illness to the patient.

One challenge of the 1980s in medical care appears to be whether a decentralized model of medical practice—family-focused, commun-ity-based, relying on integrated services delivered via a team approach—can compete with the trend towards the greater and greater corpora-tization of medicine, controlled by the largest monopolies, and ex-tending from nursing home franchises to hospital chains, emergency centers, clinics, HMOs, dialysis units, and so on. How can the doctor-patient-family relationship, so highly eulogized in medical mythology, be preserved and strengthened? Or is its demise inevitable?

The question of family therapy and counseling emerges here, too: What is the role of therapy in dealing with the many problems in liv-ing that affect families and their members, and the presence of which affect the health of millions of people? How can therapy be cost-effec-tive? How can family practice avoid a two-class system of medical care? What quality of care can be provided?

The next several years will provide answers to these questions.

TWO

What's Already Known

THEORY UNDERLYING COLLABORATIVE CARE: THE RELATIONSHIP BETWEEN ILLNESS AND THE FAMILY

A family's dynamic patterns affect both how illness arises among its members and how it is experienced. This understanding constitutes the underpinnings of contextual medicine. It embraces such factors as the likelihood of people's developing an illness—infectious, genetic-hereditary, stress-related—in a particular family context; looking at how and when a family brings or fails to bring the ill member to the physician; and analyzing different families' interpretations of illness ("attributions") and their ways of caring for their sick. Understanding family dynamics helps clarify what happens when the family caretaker (for example, the mother) herself becomes sick, when the wage earner(s) become sick, when a child—only child, eldest child, youngest child, and so on—becomes sick (compare Huygen, 1978, for an excellent description of some families in which this particular situation occurs). The links between the *familial* context (in other words, psychosocial factors that surround and condition illness—familial, cultural, occupational, religious, and so on) and illness include findings such as the increased risk of morbidity among the bereaved, especially (younger) widowers; the appearance of illness at a time of life stress, difficulties in the management of illness in a family context (compliance, relapse, ways the illness affects the family); as well as the phenomena of psychosomatic disorders and "psychosomatic families" (compare Minuchin et al., 1978).

Over the past 30 years family physicians, family therapists, and family-oriented social scientists have developed these insights. Within family medicine, the idea of seeing the family as the basic "unit of medical care" (Schmidt, 1978) has attracted a wide following, encouraging researchers to probe the ways family factors promote, prevent, or cope with stress. A rich literature has emerged on the interconnections between families and illness. Conferences and monographs have been devoted to this topic, and the journal *Family Systems Medicine* has also augmented the development of this perspective.

Fundamental to this view is the conviction that one cannot understand a patient's illness without knowing the social, emotional context in which he or she lives. Caregivers should know the family, work, school, community, ethnic, and religious aspects of the lives of the people they treat; for, when people become sick, their entire social network (or lack of one) is involved in the treatment efforts.

Although other social systems are involved in people's illness experience, the family is usually the critical unit. More than any other social system, the family defines, conditions, promotes, incites, affirms, negates, questions, softens, cares for, and otherwise creates the meaning of illness in people's lives. People live in families, become ill in families, and are treated by physicians within their family setting. Anyone concerned with contextual medicine (Worby, 1982) must look to the family as the setting for the patient's illness.

It is amazing that medicine had gone for years *without* going more deeply into the patient's family context. As Watzlawick et al. (1967) comment, "In modern biology, it would be unthinkable to study even the most primitive organism in artificial isolation from its environment" (p. 258). And yet this is precisely what medicine had done.

Exceptions existed, of course. The psychoanalysts, who were interested in childhood dynamics, occasionally provided accounts of their patients' family life. General practitioners, who dealt with families for decades and who saw the evolving patterns of illness across the generations, commented on the ways families focused around illness and on the relationship of illness and morbidity to family stress four decades ago (Richardson, 1948; Kellner, 1963); but their findings did not then excite widespread interest in a profession that was intent on specialization.

Schmidt (1978, p. 303), explaining the importance of taking the family as a basic unit of health care, noted that:

> when providing primary medical care, there seems to be a definite advantage in centering this care about the family unit rather than the isolated

individual patient. In other words, knowing what is 'going on' in the family seems to be equally as important as detailing the individual's symptoms.

He then listed several areas in which this approach seems productive: (1) the family's contribution to the "cause" of disease; (2) the family's contribution to the "cure" of disease; (3) the family's response to serious or chronic disease; and (4) the family's desire and/or need for family-oriented care.

Such a perspective rests on several assumptions: first, that emotional stress affects illness—what I call *the psychosomatic premise*; second, that symptoms, in fact all illness behavior, are understandable: their meaning emerges and becomes clearer when seen in the context in which they developed—what I call the *premise of significance*; finally, that, as an illness develops, the patient and his or her family are affected by it, and modify and modulate the illness—what I call *the 'two-way' hypothesis*. Studies have now shown these assumptions are correct, their results expanding the physician's frame of reference from a one-person field to the familial and broader social fields.

Origins of a Family Somatic Approach

I have elsewhere (Glenn, 1984) detailed the roots of the family somatic approach: the influence of psychoanalysis, the development of modern stress theory, the decades of work in psychosomatic medicine, as well as traditions of social medicine and observations through years of general practice. Here, a brief summary may be useful.

Decades ago Kanner (1948) examined the transmission of parental hypochondriasis to their children, and Goldberg (1958) and Garner and Weinar (1959) both examined family influences in the so-called psychosomatic disorders. Bruch, exploring obesity and other eating disorders (1973) added a family-oriented category to her psychoanalytical perspective.

The trend received a tremendous boost from the growth of family therapy. The group at Palo Alto's Mental Research Institute, including Gregory Bateson, Jay Haley, Don Jackson, Paul Watzlawick, and John Weakland, developed an understanding of family communication patterns which they initially applied to the symptoms of the (identified) schizophrenic (1956). They then extended this understanding to other forms of behavior. Weakland (1977) coined the term *family somatics*, prophetically declaring that all symptoms, even physical illness, could be regarded simply as behavior.

These insights led to applying a family perspective to a large number of physical illnesses. Therapists shifted from investigating schizophrenic children to working with diabetic youngsters, asthmatics, and anorexics. Soon many traditional psychosomatic disorders were being pursued from a family perspective which looked at their interactional, psychodynamic, and communicational features.

Principal among these workers were Salvador Minuchin and his group in Philadelphia. Coining the term *psychosomatic families* (1978), they showed that attention to family dynamic patterns could clarify many psychosomatic illnesses.

This line of investigation dovetailed with observations from mainstream general practice and pediatrics, which noted effects of family stress on the appearance, course, and management of illness.

In 1948 the monograph *Patients Have Families* appeared. Authored by Henry B. Richardson, a general practitioner, it reported a two-year interdisciplinary study funded by the Josiah Macy, Jr. Foundation in New York City. The group studied 15 families with the goal of understanding "the interrelation between illness and the family situation." Richardson's book included the notion of the family as a "system" and as a "unit of illness," and concluded by asking practitioners to consider "the family in all its complexities." One chapter dealt with the cooperation between psychiatrist and (medical) physician in dealing with the different aspects of illness in a family setting, an approach that now seems 30 years ahead of its time.

Fifteen years later in England, the general practitioner Robert Kellner published *Family Ill Health* (1963), a report on 346 families in a British general practice. Kellner found that (1) chronic and recurrent illness in one family member had a strong effect on the health of the others; (2) an outbreak of physical illness in one family member was commonly followed by the aggravation of a mild neurosis in another; and (3) a wife's illness followed a husband's more than twice as often as the reverse.

Kellner realized that illness in the family could lead to unhappiness, neurotic symptoms, psychosomatic illness, and even physical illness in other family members. He conjectured, too, that some visits to the doctor were occasioned by reasons other than the announced complaint, and urged physicians to be more aware of such phenomena.

Other physicians were attracted by patterns in the way some families utilized their resources. Peachey (1963), focusing on a three-year period of general practice with 25 families, showed four types of attendance patterns: (1) constant illness, (2) regular periodicity, (3) clustering, and (4) simultaneity. She hypothesized that families have definite patterns of illness, and that such patterning is characteristic of a particular family. Knowing the patterns may help guide both treatment and preventive work.

Many investigators have looked into the effects of bereavement. Over and over again, the loss of a spouse has been shown to be linked with a greater susceptibility to illnesses of all types, and to death. This seems especially true for men (Kraus and Lilienfield, 1959; Kreitman, 1964; Klein et al., 1968; Young et al., 1963; Rees and Lutkins, 1967). Much of this research is summarized in monographs by Colin Parkes (1972) and James J. Lynch (1977).

Researchers looked into the infectious diseases as well. Meyer and Haggerty (1962) found that 37 percent of streptococcal infections were associated with a form of acute stress. In addition, incidence rose in families with high chronic family stress, as compared to those with low chronic family stress. Dingle and his coworkers (1964) showed that the incidence of simple respiratory illness varies according to family relationship. More recently, Patterson (1985) has addressed the notion of chronic *strain*, rather than stress in general, as a stressor of family life.

In a now classic study, Medalie et al. (1973) found that, among men subject to arteriosclerotic cardiovascular disease, "psychosocial factors" were as significant a risk factor for developing angina pectoris as was hypertension or blood cholesterol level. The weight of psychosocial factors was greater than that of cigarette smoking in predicting the development of angina. Others have confirmed this finding. Subsequently, there has been intense discussion about the role of the Type A personality (Friedman, 1969) in the development of cardiovascular disease, especially of angina and myocardial infarction.

Psychosomatic medicine has examined the relationship between stress and illness, although it has not yet focused sharply on the family as a main source of psychosocial stress and as the main context for evolving illness (compare Lipowski et al., 1977). Recently, psychoimmunologists have begun exploring how stress affects the immune system. This has implications for understanding diseases such as allergy, cancer, many types of infections—including herpes, mononucleosis, and strep throat—as well as the autoimmune illnesses. In fact, it holds implications for every disease. The recent *Psychoneuroimmunology* (Ader, 1981) goes a long way to chart this entire field, but others such as Locke (1982) and Borysenko and Borysenko (1982) have made important recent contributions. Once the biochemical, physiological reactions can be understood, it is but a matter of time before investigators can observe families in their normal routine and assess how stress predisposes one to or promotes illness.

A major summary of the current state of scientific understanding of the interrelations between the family system and illness experience came at the January 1985 San Antonio conference "Family Systems Medicine," sponsored by the Department of Family Medicine of the University of Oklahoma. (Much of the material presented will be available in print.) The entire field is growing rapidly, and it provides for study of the "missing link" in the psychosomatic explanation—understanding the actual physical working of stress on the body.

Developments in systems theory in family medicine (Huygen, 1978; Doherty and Baird, 1983; and Christie-Seely, 1984) have moved us closer to appreciating the actual practice of what is now being called "family systems medicine"—family-focused primary care medicine which sees the diverse aspects of health and illness as they come up in the family. One of their constant common principles is the collaboration between family medicine and family therapy (compare Candib and Glenn, 1983).

THE CONTRIBUTIONS OF SYSTEMS THEORY

Practitioners and patients do not exist in a vacuum. Neither are free, independent beings. Both belong to large, complicated, and often intersecting systems whose relationship to one another is constantly changing. Foremost among these are the *family system* to which the patient belongs and the *health care system* to which the practitioner belongs.

The interaction between practitioner and patient occurs in the context of these and other systems. The relationship extends to involve large numbers of people. At any given moment, an illness that is being treated by the health care provider is being actively discussed by people within these intersecting systems, all of whom have an idea about what is "really" going on, who the patient is, what problem is being manifested, and how it should be treated.

Although many different systems are involved in illness—from the molecular level to the level of the organ system, the individual, and his or her social context—the levels that most concern the practitioner are those of the individual and the family. The relationship between patient and practitioner is often the "tip of the iceberg," extending deep into both the social and familial contexts in which both the patient and the caregiver(s) are embedded and the complex health care system, at the edge of which the physician and other caregivers are perched.

To understand the significance of this interaction, we must investigate what a "systems approach" is.

Systems Theory and a Systems Approach

Systems theory has developed in the past 30 years as a way of understanding the complex organization of the world in which we live. Spurred on by work in cybernetics that began during World War II, it deals with the wide diversity of natural and social phenomena, from the very small to the very large, from human experiences to the cold and impersonal micro- and macro-cosmos.

A system is a set of objects together with relationships among the objects and among their attributes (Hall and Fagen, 1978). Objects are another term for the parts of the system. Attributes are objects' properties. Relationships tie the system together, involving the parts in mutual interaction.

Systems can be static or dynamic, closed or open. An open system exchanges materials, energy, or information with its environment. It can thus maintain itself in spite of external stress, and it can change. Many natural systems are adaptive: they can react to their milieu in order to endure and persevere. Many natural systems also have feedback, a property which permits self-regulation of activity in response to a variety of changes (such as occurs for a heater with a thermostat, or a human thyroid gland).

Systems have certain characteristics:

1. The whole is greater than the sum of its parts. (A person is more than the sum of his or her different organ systems.)
2. Whatever affects the system as a whole affects each part. (Think of all the side effects any given medication, aimed at one particular problem, can arouse in a patient.)

3. Any change in one part affects the other parts and the system as a whole. (Any illness affects the whole patient; any illness in a family member affects the people he or she lives with.)

According to Beavers (1982), four basic assumptions fall under a systems orientation:

1. An individual needs a group, a human system, for identity and satisfaction.
2. Causes and effects are interchangeable.
3. Any human behavior is the result of many variables rather than one "cause"; simplistic solutions are therefore questioned.
4. Human beings are limited and finite. No one is absolutely helpless or absolutely powerful in a relationship.

The quality of wholeness means that the system behaves as a whole, or "coherently." The parts can only be understood in the context of the whole. The quality of independence refers to the degree of autonomy each part possesses within the whole.

Finally, natural systems form both a hierarchy and a continuum. The hierarchy of systems means that any given system may at the same time be a member of a larger system. The thyroid gland, for example, is a system in its own right, comprising its various cellular, structural, and functional properties. But it is, at the same time, a part of the endocrine system as a whole. And the endocrine system is but one organ system in the body as a whole. And so on. The continuum of systems expresses the increasing complexity of organization of natural and social systems, from the smallest cellular level to the aggregations of nations and peoples on this planet.

For further information on general systems theory, the interested reader is referred to the works of Buckley, von Bertalanffy, Ashby, Laszlo, and Hoffman cited in the bibliography.

A systems perspective focuses on the *interrelationships* among the parts, the glue that holds the system together. It examines process and the communications between the different members. It also examines how systems handle change. Some living systems become transformed over time: an acorn becomes an oak; the baby becomes an adult. A tiny town grows into a city, and then becomes a ghost town when its reason for growth recedes. An infection expands into an epidemic. An illness gives way to cure. A momentary worry becomes an all-involving obsession. This constant give-and-take between pressure for change (morphogenesis) and pressure for sameness (homeostasis) makes possible the dialectics of systems.

Systems thinking undercuts notions of simple causality, and looks instead at *what* happens rather than trying to figure out *why*. The tendency to go after the how rather than the why links it, scientifically, to the work of Claude Bernard. For, in his famous work, *An Introduction to the Study of Experimental Medicine*, he comments: "The nature of our mind leads us to seek the essence or the *why* of things . . . [but] experience soon teaches us that we cannot get beyond the *how*."

A systemic perspective describes patterns of recurrent behavior and sequences of interaction, rather than worrying about which particular piece of behavior "comes first" or "causes" the others. Systemic notions of causality have been dubbed "circular" as opposed to "linear," the implication being that systemic processes have no beginning and no end, but continue to evolve through time. Circular causality frees up any one member from being "to blame."

From this viewpoint it follows that to understand malfunction in any living system—illness, for example—one needs to grasp the system as a whole, not just one aspect.

Although the hierarchy of systems can relate to factors quite large (the ecosphere's relation to physical illness), in actual practice the physician deals mostly with the family system and its relation to the medical system.

The Family System

Each patient has his or her family system. This social unit is itself in evolution, yet we can all boast of having been born into families of one form or another, having been raised by families, and usually having the tendency to recreate the family as we move through life. The family continues to exist and evolve, and is the main social unit to which most of us belong.

Medalie (1982) defines the family as: "a group of intimate associates linked by blood, marriage, adoptive or fictive kin ties, who have mutual or common interests and activities, and who interact with each other for emotional, financial, and/or social support."

To this, we might add only that the family often has a common past and anticipates a common future.

The family is often focused around the household—people who live together—but family members hundreds of miles away may still exert a powerful influence on family life. Even deceased family members may exercise a strong influence on subsequent generations for years and years, engendering family myths and legends that are only remembered over the years and passed down from generation to generation, possessing the power to transform reality. An example of this is the alcoholic family, in which third and fourth generation alcoholics can trace their problem to a predecessor and to a family myth which they feel they have been compelled, in some helpless way, to follow.

Many theories of family life have been elaborated in recent years. Systems thinkers, especially those in the field of family therapy, have described the inner workings of the family, and have developed vocabularies to describe family patterns, the emotional and physical spaces families occupy, and the laws governing access to the dimensions of affect, power, and meaning in the family (Kantor and Lehr, 1975). Several have tried to develop a family typology (Minuchin et al., 1978; Olson et al., 1979; Fleck, 1980). Bowen (1978) has put forth a model emphasizing the three-generational development of symptoms or illness. Much of this work has been summarized by Hoffman (1981) and Walsh (1982).

Further analysis of family behavior and family dynamics is beyond the scope of this book. Suffice it to say, the family, like any other open, living system, is capable of constant change, recurring pattern, equilibrium and dysequilibrium, growth and decay. The patient is embedded in the family as a tree in the earth, and cannot be fully understood apart from it. Readers interested in further discussions of family types and family systems might consult the pages of "Family Process" and the family therapy literature.

The Health Care System

The practitioner belongs to the health care system, an enormous subunit of society involving millions and millions of people—physicians, nurses, therapists, counselors, hospital workers, clerks, paramedics, lab technicians, receptionists, x-ray personnel, and so on. This system is responsible for spending more than 12 percent of the U.S. gross national product. It extends towards other industries—the hospital supply corporations, drug companies, electronics concerns, and so on.

Patients and their families come into contact with many different health care workers in the course of their illness, any number of whom may deeply affect their lives. In the physician's office, for example, the patient or family member may become involved with the nurse, the receptionist, the billing clerk, the counselor, the social worker, receptionist, or the repairman. In the hospital, they may become involved with the nurse or orderly, the dietician, the medical student, the desk clerk, the supervisor, and the administrator.

Any of these people, meeting patients and their families, can influence the course of their disease. For example one patient's wife was told by an orderly that her husband had less than a few weeks to live, whereas the physician had said nothing like that at all. Or again, the person who sweeps the floor may stop and comment to a patient, "What? You got myeloma? Jeez, my mother had that. It's a horrible disease. . . ."

The health care system has its standards, its own codes of behavior. Coming into contact with this monolith at a time of perceived helplessness affects the patient's idea of the illness being experienced. At the same time, the health care system also restrains practitioners' behavior: physicians, for example, must be aware that other people, with somewhat conflicting interests (other generalists, specialists, utilization review committees, and the like), are looking over their shoulders. Therapists must deal with the issue of malpractice suits with reference to their potentially suicidal or homicidal patients.

Despite their vaunted independence, most practitioners are imbricated, one against the other, and jammed into a seething matrix of professional ties, rules, mores, relationships, and strains. This holds true, both for those who ply their trade "on their own" and those who are employed by others—HMOs, corporations, group practices.

The health care system itself interfaces with numerous other social systems—welfare, insurance companies, social security, legal, disability, schools, courts, and so on—in ways that draw both patient and practitioner into contact with ever-widening systemic circles.

The interrelationship of systems can be understood in the following case history:

Example: Allen F., a 35 year-old construction worker, had been seeing Dr. P. for treatment of his hypertension for many years. The physician had noted Allen to be rather high-strung, and had commented on his rather precise, obsessional manner, as well as on his seemingly sociopathic presentation. Allen F. was deferential to the point of being unctuous, and was always asking for small favors, for which he was doubly appreciative. Over time, Dr. P. learned that Allen was in a good deal of marital trouble, and that he seemed familiar with illegal drugs. Yet he had no "hard facts" to pin his observations on. Mr. F. wore an earring: What could one make of that? He lifted weights and seemed narcissistically concerned with his strength and attractiveness: What could one make of that? In addition, Dr. P. often felt physically intimidated by his patient, even though Allen F. was eternally kind and polite in his speech: What could one make of that, too? The physician felt his patient might be severely psychiatrically ill, but "compensated," but he had no evidence for this.

One day, Mr. F. appeared in the doctor's office, contrite and pleading. He had been keeping some information from the physician. Now he'd been arrested and charged with possession of narcotics. He was in a dangerous situation with the police. He had been carrying out an affair with his wife's cousin—with his wife's knowledge, he insisted— but now everything was in a turmoil. His marriage was collapsing. His "mistress" was deserting him. The police were looking to put him away. People were conspiring against him. He told of having fought the police when they came to arrest him ("I was stupid"), and of having been placed on a psychiatric ward after he "lost [his] temper." He had been given tranquilizers, but he refused to take them. It was evident that the patient had a fixed delusional system involving ideas of persecution and ideas of grandeur. At the same time he was involved in overt criminal behavior.

Dr. P. referred Mr. F. to the in-house therapist. He also prescribed a tranquilizer (Haldol) to help control the patient's violent potential. The therapist worked with the patient and his (new) girl friend, in an effort to help calm him down and help him "reintegrate." Treatment was interrupted by several court appearances. On several occasions, the patient missed sessions and stopped taking his sedatives ("They slow me down"). Finally, treatment ended when the patient, who had long before signed up with a medical HMO but had been seeing his earlier physician anyway and paying reduced private fees, announced he could no longer afford either his physicians' visits or his therapy, because he was now unemployed and had high legal bills, and he was going to get his care at the HMO treatment facility. In this manner he was lost to follow-up care.

Such an example highlights some of the systemic problems that can affect a patient-provider relationship.

A systemic approach attunes the physician to these other dimensions of the health care encounter and of the lives of his or her patient. Especially in the primary care fields, a broader perspective deepens the appreciation of why the patient has appeared and of what he or she wants, clarifies the likelihood of compliance, and hints at the significance of the encounter with the practitioner for the patient.

George Engel (1980) has provided a way for physicians to think about the different dimensions at which an illness operates. Using the example of a myocardial infarction, he shows how the patient's illness operates at the cellular level, the level of the organ and organ system, the level of the person; and how it affects the physicians, the hospital staff, the patient's spouse, the boss, and so on. He comments:

> This stands in contrast to the orientation of the reductionist scientist, for whom confidence in the ultimate explanatory power of the factor-analytic approach in effect inhibits attention to what characterizes the whole. For medicine in particular the neglect of the whole . . . is largely responsible for the physician's preoccupation with the body and with disease and the corresponding neglect of the patient as a person.

Such an approach blends the contemporary concern with the whole person with older humanistic traditions of the family doctor. It reflects the impact of social science upon medical practice and medical thought and brings practice toward a more interdisciplinary understanding.

FAMILY MEDICINE AND FAMILY THERAPY

Over the past ten years, therapists and other "systems thinkers" have been teaching family dynamics to family physicians, especially residents. They have done this as a way of addressing the question: How can family physicians understand their patients' psychosocial needs. Family physicians have been encouraged to learn basic counseling and referral skills. Several programs have used the McMaster model (Epstein and Levin, 1973; Epstein et al., 1978) to this purpose with a fair measure of success, and it is widely available to students of family medicine in Medalie's *Family Medicine—Principles and Applications* (1978). More precise intructions to family physicians have included outlines for brief therapy by the family physician (Dayringer, 1978; Bullock and Thompson, 1979) and indications for convening the family (Schmidt, 1983). Ransom and Grace (1979) have provided a thoughtful overview of the place of family therapy in family practice, and Candib and Glenn (1983) have explored some similarities and differences of the two disciplines.

The main thrust of this branch of family medicine has been to encourage family physicians to learn how to work with the family.

Working with the family (Christie-Seely, 1984) has been presented as a skill family physicians can learn, not quite so technical or difficult as family therapy. Christie-Seely distinguishes between "working with families" and "family therapy," and argues that the former lies well within the realm of family medicine. Doherty and Baird (1983) encourage family physicians to learn "primary care counselling skills," but they agree with Christie-Seely that physicians should refer patients to a friendly therapist when problems become too difficult. Much of this interest in physicians' learning counseling skills stems from Michael Balint's instructions to British GPs to work at a "deeper level" with their patients (1957), and reflects an interest in psychological process that has marked family medicine since its inception.

This challenging approach has attracted a few brave family medicine souls to therapy training, thereby creating a handful of curious hybrids. It may also have unintentionally frightened other family physicians away from working with families by intimidating them with therapy skills.

There has been an ongoing struggle in family medicine about its relationship to family therapy. Some family medicine leaders seem to want family medicine to move back closer to traditional (biomedical) medicine. Other luminaries still perceive the uniqueness of family medicine in its breadth of scope, and welcome further involvement with the behavioral sciences. At present, the fields have an uncertain alliance. Efforts are constantly being made to define each field's domain. At present, family physicians are encouraged to do primary care counseling if they wish, but the main emphasis is on physicians' learning to work with, speak to, listen to, mutually understand, and refer to collaborating therapists.

SOCIAL NETWORKS

A positive relationship exists between the supportive quality of people's social networks and such people's overall health. People with friends and families, especially ones who involve them emotionally, actually tend to live longer and enjoy better health. A recent study by Lisa Berkman and Lester Breslow (1983) provides evidence for this.

The authors were studying different health practices such as cigarette smoking and alcohol consumption. They also examined people's membership in four types of social networks and evaluated these networks as predictors of mortality over a nine-year period. They found

that people's involvement in marriage, contact with friends and relatives, church activity, and participation in other social groups were all
associated with a lower mortality. This was especially true for people
who were married and for those who had frequent contact with their
friends and relatives. It was especially true for men, less so for wom-
en. The most isolated men, for instance, had a 230 percent greater
mortality risk than the men with the strongest social connections. For
the most isolated women, the risk was 280 percent greater. These findings held firm, even when the variables of weight, cigarette smoking,
alcohol consumption, and physical activity were controlled.

The differences for men and women were interesting. For example, although having a wife seemed to be an important factor in promoting the overall health of men, being married and having a family
does not seem to function in the same way for women. Berkman and
Breslow found that never-married women actually had better health
scores than married women, and that married women without children
had better scores than those with children. This finding prompted
Joan Patterson (1985, p. 112) to wonder:

> Do married women, especially mothers, pay a price in terms of physical
> health for this type of social membership? Are these health trends related
> to the changing roles of women toward greater employment outside the
> home with no commensurate decline in household responsibilities?

Certainly, other (sociocultural) factors must be involved here. What
do women give up to maintain their marriage and/or family? Do men,
by and large, fulfill their ambitions outside of their families, and use
their families for emotional support? Where does that leave the wom-
en who are married, with families, but who do not work? The findings
lead to a multitude of questions, all critical for understanding the links
between women's family responsibilities and their health. What do
friends provide as a social support for women with children? What is
the difference between the health of working mothers whose families
support their working and that of mothers whose families criticize
their being employed? What is the difference between working-class
women and women with professional jobs? What is the role of friends
and family for women with children, and what happens to women
who lack such supports? Finally, what is the difference between the
health of married women whose husbands have traditional views of
women's work and those whose husbands tend toward a more liber-
ated view?

This latter question points to differences between subjectively perceived stress among people. Three people exposed to poverty may all react differently. So may three people exposed to the frustrations of being laid off their job, waiting for an hour in line, or facing housing discrimination. Marriage mates may share a lot in terms of attitudes toward life, but they may differ, too. What is the importance of whether the partners agree in their expectations?

Such questions naturally lead to the issue of *coherence*. Do different people's views in a family or a marriage fit with one another or not? Are people pleased with what they get in the relationship? Are they surprised? Dismayed? Outraged? Vindicated? Nonplussed? Aaron Antonovsky's writings suggest that the lack of fit between people's expectations of life and their actual experience in fact creates the (subjective) sense of stress. People who expect little from their lives may not be as stressed when they encounter hardship as are people who expect more. In fact, Antonovsky's writing suggests, the formers' psychological set and social support systems probably help them cope with their hardship. By contrast, people who expect to succeed (and whose social contacts demand it of them) can be badly shocked when they meet with adversity, for it stimulates their sense of personal failure. This type of thinking suggests a more sophisticated way of understanding the effects of stress on people's lives than simply assigning an absolute figure to different kinds of stresses and then adding up one's total. Different stresses may weigh different amounts to different folks.

Antonovsky is a sociologist who has focussed on medical issues for more than two decades. His book *Health, Stress and Coping* (1979) begins by considering the general phenomenon of health:

> Let me put it bluntly. Given the ubiquity of pathogens—microbiological, chemical, physical, psychological, social, and cultural—it seems to me self-evident that everyone should succumb to this bombardment and constantly be dying (p. 13).

How, with so many pathogens and harmful sources of stress surrounding us, do so many of us remain healthy? Pursuing this question of "salutogenesis"—the origins of health—Antonovsky postulates a health ease/dis-ease continuum, which contrasts to the sick/healthy orientation of the nineteenth century medical model. What, he asks, keeps people toward the healthy end of the spectrum?

He rejects the notion that it is the absence of stressors, for "stressors are omnipresent in human existence." Distinguishing between tension (the response of an organism to stressors) and stress (the state of an organism in response to failure to manage tensions well), he searches for a key to the successful management of stressors in everyday life. He proposes that it is a sense of *coherence*,

> a global orientation that expresses the extent to which one has a perva-
> sive, enduring though dynamic feeling of confidence that one's internal
> and external environments are predictable and that there is a high prob-
> ability that things will work out as well as can reasonably be expected
> (Antonovsky, 1979, p. 10).

Antonovsky accepts the impact of many factors on people's state of health, and his analysis has many applications in the treatment of problems in living. His view is consistent with the many studies showing links between untoward stress and disease, and also with studies showing how illness can be combatted. His findings dovetail nicely with the findings of Berkman that social support networks have a positive correlation with mortality and morbidity.

More critical than his hypothesis, however, is Antonovsky's basic stance, which is firmly against biomedicine's obsession with pathology:

> First, the pathogenic approach pressures us to focus on the disease, on
> the illness . . . and to disregard the sickness . . . the subjective interpre-
> tation of the state of affairs of the person who is ill. . . . Second, think-
> ing in pathogenic terms is most comfortable with the "magic-bullet"
> approach—one disease, one cure. . . . Third, pathogenesis by definition
> is a model that postulates a state of disease that is qualitatively and di-
> chotomously different from a state of nondisease (pp. 36-37).

The implications of such an approach are evident in the split between medical and nonmedical ways of viewing and treating stress, a split that may arise when collaborating health practitioners try to deal with the "same" problem. On the one hand, the medical model (including many schools of psychotherapy) links stress with illness; ineffective coping ties into the appearance of disease. Thus, the problem of stress is "medicalized," and so is its treatment. Those standing outside the medical model will tend to approach stress and its effects as phenomena of life: problems in living, if you will, requiring perhaps further education and training in ways of managing such stress, but not "therapy."

Antonovsky also suggests why some groups of people exposed to what seem repeated, unremitting stress do not develop scores of diseases. People who expect their lives to be hard, and whose neighbors

and families share their expectations, do not feel the same frustrations as do those who expect life to reward them to the hilt (and
"fairly").

This kind of thinking would also help explain, for example, why
a family in some instances acts as a social support, a positive influence,
and in other instances is a mainly negative factor, creating discord,
leading to dispute, and underscoring people's sense of worthlessness,
failure, and frustration. The concept of *fit* explains how we inwardly
experience things. It is a notion which collaborating health care professionals need to translate into their own disciplines, and then discuss
together.

PREVENTIVE MEDICINE

Preventive medicine has had a curious history in recent years. First
it was ignored, except in the field of public health. Then in the period
between 1960 and 1975 it was rediscovered, and health care practitioners imagined the benefits of a health system that truly cared about
prevention of disease, rather than simply treating it over and over
again. This led to attention to factors such as people's diet and nutrition, the way they managed stress, concern with factors of occupational health, the role of air and water in the promotion and/or prevention of disease (Hippocrates, revived!), the role of social class,
poverty, ghetto life. It seemed health care work was going to extend
to look at life in general, in an attempt to help create healthful en-
vironments.

Then, as the costs of pursuing all this started rising beyond anyone's worst nightmares, people began to back away from the more
global, societal dimensions of preventive health. Instead, over the past
decade, attention has been focused on two aspects of preventive medicine that still claim a good deal of attention: (1) efforts to prevent
illness because of the cost savings promised, and (2) efforts to prevent
illnesses that are within the control of the individual patient—cigarette smoking, consumption of alcohol, dietary intake of fats, wearing
seat belts when driving. (These have at times seemed part of a "blame
the patient for the disease" syndrome—especially when grouped together with physicians' and other health planners' insistence in noting
that a high percentage of the health care budget is spent caring for a
relatively few chronically ill patients. It's not clear what these folks
are implying: Should we kill the sick elderly? Should we abandon all
patients who drink more than a certain· amount a day and/or who

smoke more than two packs of cigarettes a day? Should insurance be reserved for the basically healthy?)

In all this rush toward contemporary preventive medicine, I am astounded by how few people are talking about the preventive health aspects involved in looking at health and disease from a systems perspective. This would follow the lines of hoping to save money and/or prevent illness by intervening prospectively with high-risk families, and by using counselors or therapists to treat illness conjointly with physicians, and in a family context. If you think about it, however, this train of thought follows directly from what's been learned over the past 30 years. Attention to familial factors in health and disease can save a lot of money, and it can prevent a lot of unnecessary suffering. This is part of the economic rationale for developing collaborative care, and for moving more strongly away from the specialist-oriented model. These days, however, preventive medicine is almost always *individually* oriented.

THREE

Some Basic Notions

Health practitioners use the same notions over and over, but the contexts in which they are applied constantly differ. Conditions differ from one family to another, from generation to generation, from one region of the country to another, and from nation to nation. Our notions change slowly, reflecting both our experience and the shifting reality with which we must cope. After several years, a health practitioner's ideas may evolve in a particular direction, while the reality of his or her patients' lives shift in another. For example, older practitioners, familiar with the dilemmas of parenthood, may modify some of their earlier ideas about adolescent rebellion; at the same time, their practice may include younger people who do not share this perspective.

Change is the basic constant in history. Whatever we watch changes as we watch it: becoming bigger or smaller, older or younger, smarter or more foolish. Whatever notions we consider "basic" to people's condition alter in the light of changing social conditions in the cauldron of history.

Because of this, thinking people periodically reexamine their own values and assumptions. This chapter reflects on some of the common assumptions we use every day, the significance of which is deeply involved in any attempt to develop collaborative health care.

COMMUNITY

If we are going to talk about community-based health care, we need to understand what we mean by *community*. The concept is complicated, because people use it to connote different entities, and because communities themselves have grown more complex and diverse. Especially when the term is invested with a moral tone (as in "community-based health care," where the community is a near-reverential object as well as the context of care), it is critical to understand just who "the" community is.

Traditional notions of community conjure up small-town American life in New England or the Midwest. This type of community is remarkably homogeneous: everyone holds similar values, and the people are usually white and Protestant, similar ethnically and culturally. Even where class differences exist, they have developed because there are different tasks to be done for the common good—blacksmith, farmer, teacher, banker, workhand, housewife—and people value one another's contributions to the overall whole.

Such communities tend to be small. Everyone knows everyone else, and every person has a place in the overall life of the town, whether it is the town fool, pretty young thing, bright young lad, dreamer and poet, ne'er-do-well, factory hand, den mother, or a multitude of other possibilities. This, however, is the stuff of myth and fancy. These powerful, anachronistic images are reinforced in our minds by TV programs such as "Little House on the Prairie" and by countless films and stories. They are bolstered by the recent outpouring of nostalgia for the past, especially the imagined uncomplicated life of early America. Such a notion of community is peopled with stereotyped inhabitants, such as, for example, the old family doctor (smelling of whisky and slightly overweight, clad in his white shirt, dark suit pants and vest) often driving in his car or horse-drawn sleigh to pay a house call to his sick patient. This sense of community corresponds more to people's collective fantasies and wishes for an untrammeled life than to any reality we experience together now, except in rare situations. The notion is romantic, idealistic, and sentimental. It may capture our fancy, charm us by its simplicity, and even play a role in children's images of what they want to be when they grow up and of how people in a community ought to act. Yet few of us have found such a community in which to live and practice. Communities today are more complex and change much more quickly.

Most people today actually live in a number of different communities: church group, ethnic group, occupational group, generational cohort, social class, hobby enthusiast group, and so on. One's circles can't be defined spatially as easily as they used to be. People experience interfacing communities, intersecting groups. Even the geographical community is no longer a "community," no longer the "neighborhood" of Norman Rockwell paintings. Instead, it is a place where different groups, or communities, of people live.

Talcott Parsons (1951) defines a community as "that collectivity the members of which share a common territorial area as their base of operations for daily activities" (p. 91). But reflection today will show that such a definition is inadequate. Commenting on this dilemma, Reiss and Oliveri (1983) state:

> In simpler societies, "culture" and "community" may be regarded as roughly synonymous. The prevailing standards and practices of the family's community (village, tribe, etc.) are a single-voiced expression of the prevailing beliefs and values of the culture. In more complex societies, the community is more heterogenous and, though by no means mute . . . may speak with several voices. Moreover, for highly mobile families or even for sessile families with cosmopolitan perspectives it may be difficult to define the "community" whose values and conceptions are most influential. Nonetheless, for simplicity's sake, we will define a family's community as *those social settings of its everyday life* [italics mine]. In urban settings, these will include neighborhood, major friendship and kin networks and occupational and school settings. In a complex urban setting each of these might constitute separate social worlds—perhaps with conflicting perspectives, images and values. It is important that many of them are not simply voluntary but that the family is actively recruited or coerced into some by law (school) or by need (occupational setting) (p. 66).

Not only do we belong to a diversity of communities; some of them are voluntary and others are compulsory. We are born into some communities—ethnic group, race, sex, family; join others by choice and preference—religious group, profession, hobby, marriage; and are driven into and/or choose yet others—poorer social classes, criminal life, madness.

H. Jack Geiger, in an excellent chapter in Connor and Mullan's *Community Oriented Primary Care* (1983), also faces this question of defining the community, when one's concerns are providing community health care:

> There is a major difficulty, for us, with these definitions of COPC. . . .
> We do not have regionalization of primary care, with registered patients and clearly defined populations eligible to use a specific practice, and there is no way for a single practice to 'accept responsibility for the health of a community,' in most instances, even if it wanted to. We have

multiple competing providers, selling personal health services to individuals or small groups, not communities. . . . The reimbursement system offers almost no incentive for cooperation, but many for competition. . . .

Most American communities are not anyone's defined population for medical care. Most American consumers of medical care—the term itself reflects the structure of the system—do not regard themselves as part of anyone's defined population. For most people, a sense of belonging to a community does not extend to the process of seeking medical care; there is no perception of shared risks, problems, or goals, except in the face of major environmental hazards or a widespread lack of access to care for geographic or financial reasons, or because of health manpower shortages.

A single family may regularly consult a pediatrician, an internist, and one or two subspecialists, unconnected with each other and located outside the immediate community. In urban areas, a single city block may house a thousand such families, using several thousand physicians and a dozen hospitals among them. Outreach efforts and household surveys may be seen by such families as an aggressive intrusion and an invasion of privacy; they have not decided to be part of any practice's community program (p. 72).

To this list of difficulties in defining a community for community-oriented primary care may be added the following: (1) mobility—between 1975 and 1976, 40 percent of the population of the United States moved at least once (Geiger, 1983, p. 73), which keeps changing the character of many communities; (2) the fee for service method of providing medical care which enables some people to obtain treatment while keeping others away; (3) a medical model that values technical expertise rather than a psychosocial perspective; (4) the pluralism of health care, which puts many different providers into the same community, competing for their share of patients; and (5) the prevalent view of providing health care to individuals, not groups of people (Madison, 1983, p. 122).

This dilemma has been felt acutely by many professionals concerned with providing community-oriented health care. After all, health care practitioners with a broad perspective on their work want to provide continuity of care over time; thus they need a community that perseveres, whose members are accessible for care. They want to provide care in a definable context; thus they need a community whose members—families, church-goers, school personnel—can be clearly identified. They want to work where there is a sense of community among the patients, not just among the providers; thus, they need a community whose members have "community-consciousness."

What different kinds of communities are there. *Community* can be defined as follows:

• A geographical area: essentially a catchment area. Everyone who lives in this area lives in the "community." This definition works fine for ghetto communities and ethnic communities; it even works for retirement communities and old (small) Yankee towns. It works less well for communities that are suburbs, bedroom communities, or places where people want to be alone. One problem with the simple geographic definition is that people can live close to one another, *among* one another, if you will, within easy reach of one another, and yet have very little sense of a shared community. This holds for many urban areas, where people may be neighbors but may not speak more than ten words to one another in a year: their identities are in other communities.

One issue that arose in the 1960s is, who speaks for the community? Persons frequently appeared, claiming to be spokespeople for a community, but they were not recognized as such by everyone else in the community. When people are organizing the community, or asking for community representation on an advisory board, this issue becomes a problem. Do local businessmen speak for the community? Do militant welfare mothers speak for it better? Would one involve both, or one group to the other's exclusion. Does one seek out community leaders or community representatives? People with their own ideas about things, or people who will acquiesce to what is being done "for" them? Are "leaders" self-appointed, or have they developed a following? Because geographic communities and neighborhood include a mix of people, this is always a thorny question. Who speaks for which part of the community? Who speaks for the whole?

• A like-minded, like-constituted cohort of people—people who share the same kind of religious or ethnic background (the Polish community, the Jewish community). Such ethnic communities often develop their own institutions—community centers, churches, schools, cultural groups. Depending on the intensity of coherence among its members, this can be one of the main communities people belong to. The renaissance of Jewishness among middle-class Jews is part of a current phenomenon for regaining identity through participation in the religious community. In the same vein, Polish-Americans or Italian-Americans may preserve their ethnic-cultural identity through community clubs, games, musical events, ethnic costumes, preservation of their language, celebration of national holidays, encouragement of ethnic bakeries and restaurants, and ethnic libraries. It remains to be seen how strongly these ethnic communities will survive into the twenty-first century. Many ethnic areas in large U.S. cities seem dominated by the elderly, with the younger people—as they have often done—moving out and tending toward assimilation with the larger culture and community.

• A defined neighborhood, often but not necessarily containing people of the same social class, people who share the same local concerns, who have to cope with the same social and natural environment: schools, garbage collection, stores, youths, pollution. This is similar to the first definition, but connotes a smaller more carefully delimited place. For some people, the neighborhood is their main community. They are intent on keeping property values up, on keeping crime away, on making sure that only "nice people" move in, on enforcing local laws and customs. This may be so, even when the neighborhood is quite diverse ethnically or racially, or even when its members come from different classes. The main concern here is with maintaining decent local living conditions for people in the neighborhood. In exchange for neighborhood spirit—encouraging local youths in sports, patronizing the local merchants, watching one another's children—people receive a sense of togetherness and a feeling that they are not alone in their life space.

• A spiritual group. Here we can consider cult groups, religious communities such as monasteries or nunneries, or other cliques whose members' allegiance to one another rests on their shared exclusion from the rest of society.

• A group that has its own particular local geographical and cultural identity—the Roxbury community, the South End community. Such a community can be very "tight" indeed, for it combines local boundaries with ethnic homogeneity, and adds to them the strength of several different generations of the same group all working together for the common good. Such communities often exist in poor rural areas or in urban ghetto areas, where the community's cohesive force creates a family-like spirit that offsets the bruised social connections and lack of common supports and resources that some members experience.

• Workers in a factory, students in a school, and so on. Occupational communities are quite often very strong. By their nature they exclude other members of the worker's family, but often try to make up for this by having a women's auxiliary or by instituting group/family outings. At the height of the labor movement in the United States, union members developed a sense of solidarity across trade lines, and organized spouses and families into strong support groups at times of strife and struggle. One thinks, for example, of the community of Lowell mill hands who, linked to other U.S. workers, sent their children to safer, sympathetic families in other cities during part of their strike. At the height of the protest against the Vietnam War, students formed a vast nationwide community, too. People from other schools were seen as brothers and sisters in the "Movement" against the "system." But such times do not last. When there is struggle or suffering, work and school (and class and political) ties can be intense. At other times, they can be so weak that common struggles (for example, strikes) are defeated, thus leading to demoralization of the community.

• "People registered as potential users of a physicians' group practice, health maintenance organization, neighborhood health center, or other defined service" (Abramson and Kark, 1983, p. 24). Such a definition represents a "provider's" view of community: all the people that shop at Zayre's, all the people enrolled in the Humana HMO, all the people who go to the movies. If the consumer represented in such a community is very concerned about the product or service being provided, then such a community may assume a significance in people's lives. If not, the concept is more a concern for marketing, advertising, and business than anything else. When people see themselves as consumers of medical care, as a group, then they will exercise more input in the structure of health care delivery. When not, the health care organizations will take the leads in aggressive marketing, capitalizing on the various psychological aspects of health care as perceived by their potential patients.

Just because people move doesn't mean they don't want something stable when they stop moving. Communities are usually in flux. There is a tension between the people who have been in the community a long time, the people who are getting ready to leave, and the people who have just (or are just newly) arrived. Especially in regard to medical care, these groups may have different concerns. Those who have been in the community for some time will look to the other institutions in the community, the physicians and the hospital(s). Those who are ready to leave will not have the same allegiance. And those newly entering may look for stability, or they may patronize other newcomers without roots, like themselves (such as the local Health-Stop facility).

In the past, some ethnic or union groups had looked at health care as a matter of intense community concern. The outcome of such concern was union-linked medical programs, ethnic or religiously founded hospitals—Sancta Maria Hospital, Beth Israel and Mount Sinai, Swedish Hospital. The same feelings led to community-based health clinics (neighborhood clinics) in many poor and minority areas in the 1960s.

• "Users of a defined service, or repeated users of the service" (Abramson and Kark, 1983). Once again, people who frequent a particular service or provider can be viewed as a community, both in the subjective aspect of user who wishes to shape the product or service—as with Ralph Nader's groups of concerned consumers—and in the objective aspect of consumer, as seen by the provider of such service. Such a notion of community, however, seems fairly thin today.

How does one deal with a patient and/or family's being embroiled in several different communities at once? Reiss and Oliveri (1983, p. 76) provide a clear guide: seek out the "regnant" community, the community that holds the most meaning for the involved people:

> There are two fundamental assessments that are required for delineating the [relevant] community frames. First, we must identify the community or communities in which our family holds membership. In simpler societies we may need to delineate only one such community. In more complex societies there may be two or more; one of these may be clearly regnant, as in the case of well-demarcated ethnic communities and economically privileged communities in this country. The second assessment, of course, is to define the community's frame by delineating the magnitude of importance or of expected disruption it assigns particular events, its punctuation of those events and its conception of family accountability, duty, and competence.

This seems a commonsensical approach, similar to the concept of "brightness" I have elaborated elsewhere (Glenn, 1984), which helps the overburdened professional sort out the relevant from the less relevant factors affecting the health and well-being of the people he or she is caring for.

There are thus many ways to look at a person's community. These can be split into two basic perspectives: objective and subjective. In the *objective* sense, a community is a larger social context in which an individual (or family) can be placed by any observer. This would include grouping people together by neighborhood, race, sex, age, occupation, insurance program, and so on. In the *subjective* sense, a community is a larger social context in which an individual places himself or herself. Such a definition embraces the affective ties a person has to a particular community, and designates the felt degree of belonging. It is important to consider both these perspectives, for an individual may be a member of a neighborhood by virtue of living in it, and yet have no sense of identity with that neighborhood. A person may be a member of a racial or ethnic group by birth, and yet have very different feelings about membership in that group than another person in the same family. The epidemiological approach always considers things from the *outside*. Human experience is mainly felt from the *inside*, and thus people's feelings about their own proper community must be considered as well as any epidemiological groupings done by the outsider.

THE FAMILY

Just as we feel we know what a community is, so we know what the family is, too. But the family is also in flux and transition today, and old images and definitions no longer correspond to reality. Just imagine the different ways people live these days. The extended family has almost disappeared. People live in one- and two-, not three-generational units. And yet there are one-parent families, communes, peer groups and collectives. Many people live alone, isolated from any family. Aging couples live together without children; two sisters live together, families live on one floor of a building with their parents upstairs or downstairs. Our understanding of "family" has tremendous implications for disciplines such as family medicine or family therapy, or any other family-centered discipline.

Just as with the notion of community, it is useful for us to separate the objective ways a family may be defined from the subjective ways that family is experienced. The former includes a wide number of attempts to define the family in a demographic or epidemiological sense; the latter, different ways to credit the number of individuals for which any given person has "family feelings."

Objective

I would argue that there are two main ways of objectively looking at the family. The first emphasizes kinship; the second living arrangements.

People who emphasize *kinship* look at the generations of a family (Bowen, 1978). They look at transmitted familial patterns, recurrent images and themes. The cornerstone of such an approach in family medicine is the genogram (McGoldrick and Gerson, 1985), which traces the different generations surrounding any given individual. It provides room for transcribing the incidence of family illness, family behavioral patterns, and family secrets. The underlying assumption here is, that the biological family, extending through time—the family tree—carries the most essential information about an individual's sense of family. Recursive patterns will be sought. Possible biologically linked behavioral disorders will be noted. Inherited difficulties will be given high priority. Though clearly carrying basic information, this approach carries with it a biological bias which, at times, can be dangerous, especially if not tempered by a curiosity for psychosocial surround.

The second approach is more empirical: to look at the ways in which people live, and to consider a person's family as synonymous with the household in which he lives. This must have been a simple, sound approach in earlier days, when in fact most people lived with their (extended!) families, so that kinship-family did not differ all that much from household, except that the kinship unit was larger and more extensive. Today, however, when many people live apart from almost all of their relatives, the sense of family-as-household provides a different, counter-balancing way to look at a person's "family" than the kinship view.

Ransom (1985), pursuing this view, analyzed recent census data to argue that family medicine has not kept its notions of family in line with contemporary life. Families are often conceived of traditionally, as the nuclear family—wage-earning husband, housewife-mother, and their children—while other forms of living arrangements have been ignored. If one looks at the actual living arrangements—households—in the United States, one finds a vast and heterogeneous array of ways in which people live.

About 5.8 million persons in the United States live in group living quarters, such as dormitories, barracks, prisons, and hospitals. The remainder live in households. Seventy-three percent of these households in 1980 were family households including two or more persons living together who were related by birth or marriage. This represents a decline of 8 percent from 1970, when the figure was 80 percent. Married couple households, which increased in number by 4.5 million over ten years, actually fell in percentage from 70 percent to 60 percent, while single-parent households, which increased by 4.3 million in number, increased by percentage of all households from 7 to 13 percent. This dramatically shows the rise of the one-parent (90% mothers) family today.

In addition, 27 percent of households were "nonfamily," a growth of 85 percent in a decade. Of these, 23 percent were people living alone (18 million people), and 4 percent were households of nonrelated people, people living with roommates, such as two men or two women, or a group of people living communally.

This erosion of the traditional family/household is further accelerated by the increase of double-wage-earning families today—greater than the number of one-income couple families—as well as by the number of households represented by the aging couple without children or whose children have moved away.

Ransom (1984, p. 455) comments: "Melodramatically, what comes to mind as the traditional nuclear family—a breadwinning father, a housewife mother, and two children under 18 at home—accounted for only 5% of households and only 8% of all couple families in 1981."

Using this data, Ransom argues strongly against the romanticized image of the nuclear family as constituting "the" family. Such a view implies that this type of arrangement is the preferred, normal, or usual family, and yet such is neither the case in actual fact, nor is it automatically the best way to live:

> The problem with the traditional nuclear family idea for medical practice is that it is both value-laden and unrepresentative. As the numbers show, it is only one in a spectrum of social forms in which people live today, and a diminishing one at that, demographically speaking. When family practice training and family physicians' offices are organized with the goal of serving nuclear families in mind, trouble is bound to enter (1984, p. 455).

The changing family also affects the long-standing discussion in family medicine about the family as the object of medical care. Ransom (1983b) has argued that the family cannot be the "object" of care, but is the context in which care takes place. He also points out that the rise in different types of living arrangements implies that family practitioners cannot automatically assume that the nuclear family is the context of their care. Rather, they have to inquire about the actual living arrangements of their patients and proceed accordingly.

Moreover, some actual arrangements may not show up in the statistics. A married couple living in the same building as one of their parents may be living as a couple, but they are close to being an extended family. Some people's parents are next door or across town; others are in another state, across the country, or dead. Some people never leave the neighborhood in which they grew up, and have dozens of long-standing friends and relatives whom they see every month. Others live all by themselves in communities, often made up of people like themselves, uprooted and detached from their original families. Still other people live near their families but do not see them, while others, who live in another town, see their families quite often. Clearly, the problem goes beyond demographics and depends on felt ties between people.

The dichotomy between the two approaches can be likened to the old familiar discussions about Nature versus Nurture. Clearly, the "truth" is affected by both these factors—the patterns of the generations (heredity) and the immediate context of one's household.

Subjective

A person's sense of family goes beyond demographics. It rests within one's mind and memory. The sense of family includes remembrances from childhood—family gatherings, holiday meals, celebrations, and special occasions, as well as the built-up sense of daily family life—arguments with a sibling, bedtime routines, parents' habits. A sense of family also includes internalized images of family space—geography of important places, settings within one's house and room—and the internalized rhythm of family time—family speech patterns, times for preparation, waiting, the punctuation of events.

The people one counts as (real) family may vary among members of the same family. For instance, my Aunt Sunny is a clear-cut member of my father's family, because she is his sister. But as I have virtually never seen her, she is not someone I would think of when defining my own family. Other people may consider a long-deceased relative, after whom, let us say, they have been named, as an important family figure. To others, some family figures who are alive and kicking may be outside their sense of family members they think of.

The family is frequently focused around the household, especially when children are young. But as children grow older and move away, their sense of family moves out with them—although they may not keep it as intensely as their parents do. Important family members may live hundreds of miles away and still exercise a powerful influence on family life. A "matriarch," 90 years old and living in a nearby nursing home, may nonetheless still be the most important person in her family, in terms of setting values, making decisions, and approving or disapproving of one or another course of action. Deceased family members may exert an influence on subsequent generations, especially in families with a strong sense of tradition, and they may be pivotal figures in critical family legends and myths, whose deeds provide a model for their descendants. Workings of such a process can be intuited in the Kennedy family; on a less majestic level, links to past generations can often be found among the families of alcoholics.

The subjective side of "family" involves the different kinds of affect a person invests in family members, whom he or she considers close and whom distant. Which family members are positive role models; which negative ones? Which "family ghosts" continue to haunt one even into the fourth and fifth decades, and further? Which family patterns are felt to be inevitable, inviolable, invincible? Usually, such information is not sought out by most family practitioners. It is too intimate for most to grope for, and practitioners frequently don't have the time or haven't established the degree of closeness necessary to let them inquire about their patients' affective ties, their dreams and fears, their childhood memories, their models. Instead, this material has been ceded to the therapists and psychoanalysts, to make of it what they will. And yet one cannot help remarking that the greater motivations to our behavior, whether they be around our sicknesses or any other aspect of our lives, stem from feelings and values which are not clearly conscious to us, and which can be traced to deep-rooted influences which have accrued over the years.

I am not here saying that family practitioners *should* investigate such material. I fear that the great majority have neither the training, the inclination, nor (like myself) the time to pursue such curiosity. There is, after all, a limit to how deeply one can get to know a patient or client in the time allotted. What I am saying, though, is that the practitioner has to realize the importance of the subjective aspect of how life is experienced, how people behave in public, how people make decisions, how people treat one another, and how people think of themselves.

The practitioner encounters a patient's family in many ways. Family members seem to have an unlimited capacity for materializing around a crisis. They will travel hundreds of miles to be at the bedside of an ailing relative. They will phone the physician to offer advice, criticize what's being done, present a family secret which has bearing on the matter at hand, offer their own view of what the problem really is. Families can suddenly evaporate, split up, and reassemble, create subgroups, hide one of their members from society, expel someone, and so on. Many families have a "hidden patient," whose problems are not brought to the health practitioner but whose disability affects the others critically. In order to cope with such a torrent of material, practitioners need to be aware of the subjective aspects of people's sense of family; because otherwise they will act as if things are a lot more rational and decipherable than they really are.

In summary, then, the sense of family includes both objective and subjective factors. The sociology of the family is complex and changing. Practitioners who deal with people in their social and familial contexts will try to see the particular ways their patients and clients understand their family, not how they fit or do not fit into some preconceived view of family they carry themselves. Only such an open-minded approach will work in the diverse practice settings and diverse communities in which we find ourselves today.

THE PATIENT

There has been much discussion about who the patient is in any primary care discipline. The traditional position has been that the individual patient in the doctor's office is "the" patient. Any further extension is unwarranted and can be considered an intrusion beyond the doctor-patient relationship. Advocates of this view point out that only the patient has contracted for the physician's services, and the physician must respect this.

This view, can run into difficulties, however, as when the identified patient is a child, feeble-minded, senile, or damaged by virtue of illness so as to be unable to make his or her own decisions. In such instances, the traditionalists turn to the responsible family member.

Even then, however, problems arise. What happens when irate parents bring a sullen teenager for treatment, claiming that the child's behavior is a problem upsetting the family, but the teenager angrily complains that her parents are the problem. Or what happens when, faced with a dying parent, adult children disagree over who the responsible family member is, and barrage the physician with contradictory demands—resuscitate, do not resuscitate. At these and other moments the traditionalist becomes stymied and is thrown into the fires of systemic conflict.

But it is not only boundary-stretching situations that bring about a critique of the traditional approach. This approach has also drawn fire from those with insights into family dynamics, who argue that the concept of the patient always goes beyond the individual in the physician's office. If the patient's complaint is seen in its full context, then family (and other important social linkages) are always relevant.

Does this then make the family into the patient or does society become the patient . . . or what?

Family medicine has seen a decade-long debate over whether the "family is the [basic] unit of medical care." Schmidt (1978) argues for this position. In ensuing years, Carmichael (1983) and Marinker (1982), although from different perspectives, argued against considering the family as a "unit of care," that is, as the patient—even though they agreed with the notion of situating the individual patient in his or her family context; and Ransom has written extensively in several issues of *Family Systems Medicine* (see Bibliography) against what he considers simple-mindedly perceiving the family as "the patient" rather than as a key context in which health care can be provided. Ransom feels, with Carmichael, that the "family" in family medicine must be taken metaphorically, to describe the relationship between patient and physician, as well as to focus on how the individual patient fits into his or her family dynamic patterns. But he argues strongly against reifying the family, as if it had a view or could think or be sick. Such mechanistic approaches to family medicine only confuse the problem by creating a construct as "patient" that does not exist. (The family as a whole virtually never presents to the practitioner—as it does in Pirandello's *Six Characters in Search of an Author*—asking to be considered as an entity in its own right.)

Clarity on this matter is important. Insights into links between illness experience and family dynamics make it clear that the family as a social unit must command our respect and consideration. At times, the practitioners are asked to make decisions that affect the well-being of a number of family members; at times they are asked to choose between the well-being of their individual patient and that of others in the family. How they respond will echo their ethical and moral values, as well as the risks and benefits of the available options. The ubiquity of conflict will not yield to wishes for simplicity in the patient-physician relationship; and antagonisms between patient and practitioner— as when a patient demands pain-killers—and between family members and the practitioner—as when some family members insist on hospitalization and neither the physician nor patient deem it advisable—are inevitable and difficult.

All practitioners must decide again and again just who they are treating, and toward what end.

THE EXPERT

Traditionally, the practitioner has been felt to be the expert. The patient used to say, "Doc, if I knew what was the matter, I wouldn't be here," and "You tell me what to do, Doc, and I'll do it." Now the middle-class patient has become a lay expert, and arrives in the practitioner's office with a list of questions, citations from the *New England Journal of Medicine*, and a ready request for a second opinion. Furthermore, some segments of society have decided that "Medicine"—physicians in particular, hospitals especially, most medications, and health professionals in general—is "bad for their health." Thus they place the practitioner and themselves in a paradoxical position. On the one hand, they come to the "expert" for treatment, but on the other hand they deny that the practitioner is an expert at all and instead set themselves up as experts in their own right.

Much of this can be understood as conflicting styles of medical practice. Some physicians and some patients prefer what can be called the "authoritative" style of practice (Szasz and Hollander, 1956). This is the traditional style, in which the practitioner is the acknowledged expert and the patient/client follows instructions. Other patients and physicians believe that a more shared, collateral style of practice is better. With such a style of practice, the practitioner expertly advises the patient, but they make important decisions together.

Whatever the style being practiced, however, it is important that the patient and the practitioner share expectations and beliefs about the rules guiding their encounter. If a physician wants to get *off* the pedestal, but his patient wants him *on* it, there will be problems. Similarly, a physician who wants his authority to reign untrammeled will have a lot of trouble with today's well-read and inquisitive middle-class patients—and God help him if, hell-bent to do what he wants, he makes a "mistake."

WHAT IS THERAPY?

Every encounter, every interaction, every intervention has its consequences. They may be beneficial, harmful, or neither. It is impossible, however, *not* to have some effect. This holds true in the doctor-physician interaction, as in any other human encounter. Every patient encounter has some level of therapeutic effect. In this broadest sense, all medical practice is therapy of sorts.

I begin from this perspective, that medical practice is a form of human interrelatedness. It therefore has a therapeutic aspect. It may differ from other such forms, but its similarities with them overweigh its differences. Insofar as all human interaction is therapeutic (or anti-therapeutic), so is medical practice.

Physicians and researchers have documented the "placebo effect," which stems from the trust the patient puts in the physician and from the physician's aura. In this sense, too, all medical practice has a therapeutic aspect.

Usual ways of defining *therapy* focus on its being an applied skill used to help people cope with unpleasant feelings, difficult situations, or unrewarding patterns of behavior. Many forms of therapy exist; and there are many therapeutic schools, each with its own analysis, approach, techniques, and so on. Mystification of simple therapy techniques through the use of mumbo jumbo therapy jargon and guild-like arrogance have functioned to keep its simple "secrets" from the public.

If we see therapy as basically a process of human interrelatedness, then disputes between therapy schools pale. Therapy's basic quality is its healing influence on people. Thus, we can call the patient's experience with the physician therapy, just as we call the patient's experience with the therapist therapy.

This does not mean we denigrate therapy skill or assume that there is little to be learned. To the contrary, much can be learned; much, too, cannot be learned, but must come with a native empathic sense of people's suffering.

I say this in the belief that therapy, like medicine, has been *mystified* beyond belief. Focus has been on therapy as a profession, as a skill, and as a mystery. Disputes have gone on about whether family practitioners are capable of doing therapy or whether what they do with patients has to be called something else—"working with families" (Christie-Seely, 1984; Schmidt, 1983) being the most common term used. This word play has obscured the common work both therapist professionals and medical professionals do with patients, and has unhelpfully emphasized the skills each must possess rather than their common activity.

Does the family physician do the same kind of therapy as the "real" therapist? Some (Christie-Seely, 1984) hold that family physicians, mainly "work with families," an activity that is not actually family therapy. A very few family physicians, having spent the time to become specially trained in family therapy theory, skills, and techniques can legitimately be granted equal competence and stature as the therapists. These are the hybrids who attempt to bridge the field today.

Some family physicians work with a therapist in their practice (Doherty and Baird, 1983). They are less concerned, it appears, with the name of what they do than with the fact that they are doing it and making it available. It is fairly obvious, of course, that family therapists in a general medical practice will do a good deal of brief therapy and assessment, and not so much intensive long-term therapy with their clients.

Some physicians claim they can do "therapy" on their own. It is difficult to understand whether this view reflects "physician chauvinism" (physicians can do anything and therapy skills are essentially simple) or a deeper commitment to master counseling skills for the benefit of patients. There may be as many "answers" to the question as there are physician-therapists. In my opinion, what you call it is not a critical question. Turf disputes should not prevent people's getting needed help. Obviously therapy skills can be learned. And obviously, some people are more natively attuned to such skills than others. What kind of therapy is useful in a medical practice would be a more appropriate question to ask.

Every Illness Has Its Psychosocial Surround

Body and mind exist in the same person. People live in social contexts—families, workplace, neighborhoods. We all have feelings about our bodies, our health, sickness, and so on. Each visit to the physician brings elements of the patient's world—inner feelings and thoughts, images and memories; family myths and rituals (Glenn, 1982); meanings and values—into contact with the patient's medical entourage.

But each illness exists in a psychosocial context. The context affects the illness, and the illness affects the context. When one examines the overall picture, sometimes one aspect, sometimes the other, is predominant. As Don Bloch (1983) points out, when a restaurant patron is choking on a bit of food, the Heimlich maneuver is called for—immediately. The patron's family eating habits are beside the point.

·Not so the case of the teenage anorexic, whose weight loss and failure to eat are usually deeply rooted in family imagery, family conflict, and multi-generational family patterns.

The physician's task is to weigh the psychosocial and the biomedical factors involved in any given situation at any particular time and, based on such a consideration, to develop a plan of treatment. As Huygen has pointed out (1978), the family physician is often a contributor to the patient's "somatic fixation" rather than an assistant in helping the patient to reach beyond it. In family practice, the physician has multiple, repetitive opportunities to assess the role of the psychosocial context, at whatever depth or level he or she can get at it. If an intervention or interpretation is unsuccessful at one time, it can always be repeated. So long as the patient remains with the practice, the chance is always there. In the meantime, the family physician helps the patient deal with the physical problems the patient is prepared to deal with. One cannot insist patients do otherwise. One must take them as they are, trying always to share a bit of the understanding—perhaps we should say *test* a bit of the understanding—that we (think we) have.

Example: Sara A. was a 78-year-old woman obsessed with her bowels. She had been diagnosed as having irritable bowel syndrome, which later dovetailed with a developing mild diverticulosis. She was obviously depressed, but refused to discuss her feelings. Instead, each visit was focused around whether she had been having diarrhea in the past two or three weeks, or whether she had been constipated. She frequently alternated between the two, and when she was constipated she took cathartics, and when she was having diarrhea she took antidiarrheals. This was so in spite of the physician's attempt to set a simple and firm, predictable regime.

For two and then three years, Sara A. kept coming in for her visits, querulous, unhappy, grousing, and talking only about her diet and bowels. The physician inquired time and again about her family, her loneliness, her other occupations and interests—to no avail. One day, however, she mentioned in passing that her grandson's wife had just had a miscarriage, at five months, and that both she and the grandson were sorely upset and very withdrawn. She responded readily to the invitation to talk about this upsetting event, and to try to figure out, with the physician's help, what she could properly do about it to help both of them deal with it. From that point on, her visits to the office

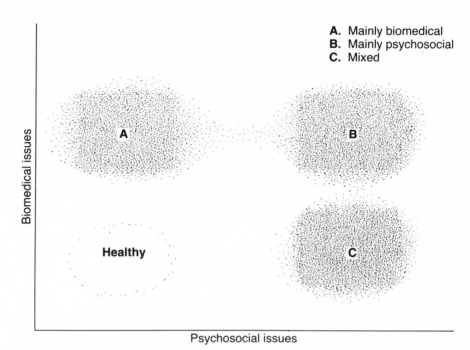

Figure 3.1 Clusters: Biomedical/Psychosocial issues.

seemed much more "human," and the content of the discussions became broader than just the state of her bowels.

One could draw a grid showing the relative weights of the biomedical vs the psychosocial factors in any patient's presentation (Figure 3.1). Some illnesses will thus emerge cast mainly in biomedical garb (acute myocardial infarction, cancer of the ovary, emphysema).Others will seem mainly emotional or psychiatric (depressive reaction, schizophrenic reaction, drug abuse). And others still will seem a sincere blend of both factors, so intertwined that they cannot be separated (childhood asthma, irritable bowel syndrome, tension headaches). Such an appraisal can help the physician to better approach the patient, the illness and the family, and draw up a strategy for therapeutics.

Some physicians may always see patients in the same category, of course. Others may develop the flexibility to understand that today Mrs. Jamison may be coming in with an upper respiratory infection. Tomorrow she may present again, worried that her daughter is sick, too. Next month she may come in vaguely fatigued, depressed because her husband has lost his job. And the next month she may come in trying to get a welfare physical form filled out, with no biomedical complaints. People can move from place to place on the graph. Astute physicians must understand this, and must constantly shift their own efforts to find just where the patient is coming from.

At times the physician may think he or she is carrying out therapy, but the patient is not in on the game. Usually, when people talk about therapy, they are referring to a conscious agreed-upon activity, with a clearcut structure, with well-defined goals, and so on. But what of the occasion when the therapist/physician thinks he or she is carrying out therapy, and the patient does not. There are four positions.

	Physician Acknowledges	Physician Does Not Acknowledge
Patient Acknowledges	Therapy	Unwitting Therapy
Patient Does Not Acknowledge	Covert Therapy	Usual Medical Practice

If one is going to work with patients, one should know at what position on the grid the encounter is taking place.

Therapy Is Always Possible

All living things undergo change. Change produces stress. Stress calls for continued adaptation. In human relationships, all of us deal constantly with stress and strain, change and adaptation.

In its most basic form, therapy is helping people deal with problems in living (Sullivan, 1953). Although we might tend to think of therapy as mainly for very sick people, this is not the case. In fact, many different kinds of people can benefit from talking to a therapist. The question should be: When is it advisable *not* to talk to a therapist? For if we are all in the process of change, and if change can produce painful dislocation, it may always be helpful, theoretically, to talk to a therapist. Reasons not to might include (1) not having the money, (2) feeling one can manage the problem one's self, (3) mistrusting therapy in the first place.

After all, most people have a number of people whose job it is to minister to their needs: the milkman, the plumber, and the electrician are a few at the workingman's level; the teacher, the priest, and the physician are some at the professional level. But very few families have a therapist they can call on when they need to. Why is this the case? It might conceivably be just as helpful to have this person at one's beck and call as any of the above-mentioned folks.

There's a lot to say about this position, both good and bad. The bad comes from the tendency to medicalize all of life. Whatever painful times we are having, there will be a medical name to fit it: a disease that describes it—menopause, depression, retardation, painful periods, pregnancy, hyperactivity, alcoholism, antisocial behavior—and a treatment held appropriate for it. The endless lists of psychiatric and psychological terms carry a deadness with them, categorizing and labeling people. So it may not, in this sense, be a good thing for people to run to a therapist whenever a problem in living emerges. It may not be good, if people think of emotional difficulties and of stress as sicknesses.

If, however, people are a bit more sophisticated, and realize that going to a therapist doesn't put them into a box, but may in fact help them get out of a box, then there's a lot to be said for making the therapist more available to more people. This only holds, however, if therapy is seen as a form of human interrelatedness, and not as some mysterious kind of treatment for an equally mysterious disease.

<u>FOUR</u>

What's Already Been Tried: Antecedents

Few people today know the rich tradition of collaborative work, and yet elements of collaborative health care have been with us, now rising, now falling, for hundreds of years. This and the following chapter present the history of earlier efforts to provide collaborative community- or family-centered health care. This chapter will focus on antecedents of such care. Chapter 5 deals with trends in collaborative care from 1945 to the present.

PHILOSOPHICAL UNDERPINNINGS OF A SYSTEMIC APPROACH

The Hippocratic Tradition

The philosophical underpinnings of a systemic perspective have been with us ever since Hippocrates. This tradition embodies both a contextual and a naturalistic approach and thus considers illness in its broader context. From its origins, the philosophy has been to include both social and physical factors in consideration. The Hippocratic tradition views disease in relationship to people's environment: food and drink, the air, weather, climate, the emotions:

> I think a physician must know, . . . about natural science, if he is going to perform aught of his duty, what man is in relation to foods and drinks, and to habits generally, and what will be the effects of each on each individual. It is not sufficient to learn simply that cheese is a bad food, as it gives a pain to one who eats a surfeit of it; we must know what the pain is, the reasons for it, and which constituent of man is harmfully

affected. . . . Cheese does not harm all men alike; some can eat their fill
of it without the slightest hurt. . . . Others come off badly. So the con-
stitutions of these men differ. . . (Hippocrates, pp. 53-55).

Whoever wishes to pursue properly the science of medicine must
proceed thus. First he ought to consider what effects each season of the
year can produce; for the seasons are not at all alike, but differ widely
both in themselves and at their changes. . . . He must also consider the
properties of the waters; for as these differ in taste and in weight, so the
property of each is far different from that of any other. Therefore, on
arrival at a town with which he is unfamiliar, the physician should examine its position with respect to the winds and to the risings of the
sun. . . . and how the natives are off for water, whether they use marshy,
soft waters, or such as are hard and come from rocky heights, or brack-
ish and harsh. The soil too, whether bare and dry or wooded and watered,
hollow and hot or dry and cold. The mode of life also of the inhabitants
that is pleasing to them, whether they are heavy drinkers, taking lunch,
and inactive, or athletic, industrious, eating much and drinking little
(Ibid., pp. 71-73).

The breadth of this perspective influenced Western medicine for
hundreds of years. For centuries, physicians sought for the fit between
people's illnesses and their way of living. The Hippocratic tradition
reigned, especially through the writings of his follower Galen, and his
influence was still strong in nineteenth century Europe before the germ
theory of disease took hold. In fact, as Dubos notes,

Until late in the nineteenth century disease has been regarded as resulting from a lack of harmony between the sick person and his environment; as an upset of the proper balance between the yin and the yang,
according to the Chinese, or among the four humors, according to Hippocrates (Dubos, 1979, p. 101).

Dubos notes that when the theory of the specific etiology of disease—the theory that germs caused diseases, that diseases had a particular offending cause—appeared in the late nineteenth century, many
physicians opposed the reductionism inherent in this view. Pidoux,
Pasteur's opponent, asserted before the Paris Academy of Medicine
that disease "is the common result of a variety of diverse external and
internal causes . . . bringing about the destruction of an organ by a
number of roads which the hygienist and the physician must endeavor
to close" (Dubos, p. 118). The older physicians combined an approach
to illness that focused on broader factors—social, psychological, physical—but their dedication to the notion of disease as "disharmony" was

unable to compete with the crisp preciseness of Pasteur and Koch's theoretical advances.

And yet the nineteenth century saw theories and discoveries that helped elaborate what is now called a "systems approach." Darwin's theories of evolution argued that species which survived had to adapt themselves to the external environment; and Claude Bernard's discussion of the "milieu interieur" held that the survival of any organism depends upon "a constant interplay between the internal and the external environment" (Dubos, p. 119). To this, Dubos comments: "The dual concept of fitness to the external environment and fixity of the internal environment is the modern expression of the Hippocratic dictum that health is universal sympathy" (p. 119).

The logical bent of the contributions is, that illness must be understood in a broader, systemic way.

The Tradition of Social Medicine

There is another trend in the collaborative approach to health and disease. Building on the Hippocratic, naturalistic tradition, writers in the nineteenth century began to move from an individual to a social viewpoint. Affected by the effects of the Industrial Revolution on the health of working people, they developed traditions of social medicine and public health that prevail today. There was a social basis for and an interest in this work, as employers wished to preserve the health of their workers to guarantee an adequate supply of labor. In addition, humanitarian considerations made those who saw the suffering of masses of working people look for solutions to the widespread, comprehensive problems of disease.

Friedrich Engels, writing in the 1840s about the condition of the working class in England (1973), pointed out the role of deteriorated social conditions on people's health. Industrial toxins polluted people's air and water supplies. Infectious diseases spread through crowded living conditions and poor ventilation. Alcoholism stemmed from poverty, stress, and exhaustion. Noise and the lack of privacy also affected people's health, as did inadequate nutrition, especially among children. Engels even analyzed the incidence of accidents—falls, drowning, and burns—among working-class children and linked this to the lack of parental presence occasioned by both parents working in the mills. Finally, Engels described specific occupational illnesses (such as miners' lung and pottery workers' lead poisoning) and linked them to people's work. His solution to these problems was a far-reaching overhaul of the power relations of society.

Dubos (1979, p. 148) notes that the idea that disease was occasioned by dirt, want, and pollution led to different trends in social medicine. One was a movement for restoring clean air, pure food, healthy water, and more pleasant surroundings. Called The Health of Towns Association, it was led in England by the physician Southwood Smith and the engineer Edwin Chadwick. It drew upon the moral fervor of the utopians, and aimed at redressing the wrongs caused by abysmal living conditions. Some of its energy led into the public health movement, sanitation, and other health reforms. The same type of movement occurred elsewhere in Europe and the United States.

Engels' writings were influential all across the continent. One physician he influenced was Rudolf Virchow, who was also beginning to view diseases as a social problem. Virchow was deeply stirred by witnessing at first hand the 1847-1848 typhus epidemic in Upper Silesia, a chronically poor area of Eastern Prussia. By early 1848, thousands were dying from hunger and the disease. Virchow travelled to the area for first-hand observation, in his capacity as a pathologist. He noted the effects of poverty, poor diet, hunger, and inadequate housing on the progress of the disease. In doing this, Virchow approached the epidemic from a systemic perspective. He noted how malnutrition predisposed to disease and how crowded living conditions also helped it spread. As Waitzkin has summarized (1981, pp. 84-85),

> Virchow noted that the overall material conditions of life created a substratum in which either health or illness flourished. He argued that economic insecurity and political disenfranchisement were, through a complex chain of causality, social problems that generated disease, disability, and early death. Economic stability and active political participation by the poor, in Virchow's view, were necessary for good health. . . . Because he saw the origins of ill health in societal problems, the most reasonable approach to epidemics was to change the conditions that permitted them to occur.

Thus, Virchow, like Engels, linked workers' illnesses to the effects of the Industrial Revolution. His solution led to increased attention to public health measures, but because he saw disease as the result of social and economic forces, his approach to public health was increasingly political. As medicine became enraptured with the theory of specific etiology of disease, Virchow's political/medical writings gradually fell out of favor.

The Health Center in the United States

In the United States, a number of different community health ventures emerged in the second half of the nineteenth century. Almost all of these were in the realm of health screening and health education, for historically the private sector opposed any public health measures that attempted to compete with its own services. The growth of health centers was permitted by the medical establishment so long as they served a strictly preventive function: "No prescriptions given, and no sickness treated" (Health Units of Boston, 1933, p. 24).

In the latter part of the nineteenth century, problems of malnutrition and infectious disease abounded in poor communities, and there were few resources to treat them. Initial efforts at providing more comprehensive health care for the poor came from such programs as the milk depots, settlement houses located in the immigrant slums, and the formation of clinics by voluntary organizations such as those concerned with infant feeding, tuberculosis, or venereal disease (Candib, 1968). Candib notes that many of these programs "were rooted in the Progressive belief in the voluntary principle and in the faith of the possibility of reforming society" (p. 7). In a similar vein, the first community health center clinics were formed in the last years of the nineteenth century. Socialist idealism and moral concern for the effects of poverty on people's welfare helped develop these measures, and they undertook to deal with disease in its social and economic setting.

A health center movement (Davis, 1927) developed between 1910 and 1915 in the large cities of the United States. One impetus to this movement was the urge to consolidate and coordinate the then existing disparate community health services. Over time, there was a gradual movement from an emphasis on progressive ideology and social commitment toward a concern with greater efficiency of organization and greater professional of care:

> The health center movement developed as the administrative response of professionals to the disorganization, duplication and spontaneity inherent in the volunteer philanthropic efforts concerned with health. It is consequently not surprising to find that the basic thrust of the health center literature is not humanitarian concern, but rather an overwhelming demand for administrative efficiency and bureaucratic streamlining (Candib, 1968, p. 8).

Michael M. Davis, chief theorist and proponent of the health center movement, cites two "root ideas" to this movement: the idea of coordination (all services in one place) and the idea of a district (all inhabitants of one area being served at one health center). As the Progressive era wound down, the city health centers sought a more professional character. Efficient operation became a methodological goal, and professional training and division of labor became more important for the health workers. As Candib notes, "Startlingly, health center literature on the whole was almost devoid of any humanitarian avowals. . . . The movement communicates no sense of immediacy about sick people, unlike the tuberculosis and infant and child health movements which had spawned it" (1968, p. 16).

Candib identifies four main tenets of the health center movement: (1) the district idea, which sought to decentralize health care services and thus make them more available, more accessible to people within the local district; (2) the coordination idea, which sought to bring all services together under one roof, thereby making the center both more efficient and more rational; (3) the 100 percent idea, which sought to register everyone in the community district and to have full community participation in the program; and (4) the generalization idea, which sought not only to bring all services together in one place, but to have all needed services available. The guiding notion was that one central clinic could provide basic health care services to an entire population within its area, thus fulfilling health concerns in an efficient manner. Many innovations were developed to meet this goal. Neighborhood health workers were trained as aides to do outreach and home visits, so that no family in the community would be beyond the center's reach. Neighborhood residents were, in some cases, brought onto advisory positions on the health center boards.

The dominance of the idea of efficiency, however, soon began to change the identity of the health centers. Efficiency became synonymous with goodness, an end in itself. Bureaucrats and professionals moved into leading positions in the health center structure. People with irregular attendance patterns were dropped from the rolls. Health professionals appeared to take greater and greater interest in their own particular roles, and the cooperative spirit began to flag. Notions remarkably similar to our current concern with cost-effectiveness appeared, and were used to justify realignment of services, paring of unproductive services, and reorganization.

Here and there exceptions rose and flourished. Wilbur C. Phillips, who had been secretary of the New York Milk Committee, began a health center in Cincinnati in 1917 sponsored by the National Social

Unit Organization. This center tried to combine both democracy and efficiency. It began as an infant and prenatal clinic, then expanded to offer medical examinations for adults, preschool children and patients with tuberculosis. Services were closely tailored to the community, vigorously pursuing the 100 percent idea, and Phillips elaborated the idea of a "social unit" which involved the community's participation in the actual governance of the health center. Such experiments sound strikingly like earlier forms of the Peckham Experiment (see below).

Similar efforts at the same time in history can be found in the history of some union health programs, whereby unions purchased health care for their members at reduced stipends from physicians who welcomed the guaranteed income.

Following World War I, the health center movement went into decline, even though there was increased interest in health in the immediate postwar period. The Red Cross, faced with the prospect of demobilizing its structure after the war, had the idea of using its resources to establish a nationwide network of community health care centers with a mainly educational orientation, but that idea failed to gather support. In addition, the increasing professionalism of existing community health centers had the untoward effect of isolating the centers from the people of the very communities they had been intended to serve.

In the 1920s the idea of model "health demonstration projects" sponsored by wealthy foundations emerged, an idea that endures in the health care field to this day. But the health centers as such dwindled and collapsed. Various reasons have been given for this. In the main, the centers were estranged from their communities and failed to garner local support and local participation. In addition, the medical establishment, which found increasing numbers of patients capable of paying for private services, opposed the community clinic concept. Their view was that public health facilities should provide only preventive and educative functions, following the slogan "No prescriptions given, no sickness treated" (The Health Units of Boston, p. 24). Many of course opposed even these functions, seeing them as taking away their own potential income. Other factors contributing to the demise of the health centers include leadership and staffing problems, difficulties with funding, and the growth of the city hospitals that could provide free health care services to city residents. In addition, some of the more radical health programs were denounced as socialistic (Stoeckle and Candib, 1969).

The Peckham Experiment

Several important collaborative health programs took place between 1920 and 1945. The Peckham Experiment in England was one which provided complete health care to a large self-selected community and which has served as an inspiration to many people in the field ever since.

In the mid-1920s, a group of social scientists and naturalists, observers of the human condition, had the "'hunch' that health was the factor of primary importance for human living" (Pearse and Crocker, 1943, p. 11). After reflecting on their convictions, they decided to offer a health service to families "constituted on the pattern of a Family Club, with periodic health overhaul for all its members and with various ancillary services for infants, children and parents alike" (p. 11), but they were not sure that people, given this opportunity, would take it. In 1926, they opened the initial Pioneer health center. It was a small house in South London, with a consulting room, receptionist office, bathroom, and club room. Families in the vicinity were invited to join for a modest weekly fee. By the end of three years, 112 families, or over 400 people, had enrolled. The sponsors felt that their initial question had been answered: people were willing to join in such a project. But they had learned something else. Although many of their initial members had not been ill, their overall "health and vitality" (p. 12) was low. The Peckham sponsors felt it was pointless to evaluate people's health through regular "overhauls" and then return the people to the same environment from which they had come. They felt that people's environment had to be more supportive of their health. It had to provide social and physical "tools" with which people could develop healthier lives. But the families enrolled in the Peckham health center lived impoverished lives. They had wretchedly few resources for growth and development. The sponsors therefore decided to close down the center and reconsider their efforts.

Peckham's founders believed that human beings had a biological potential for healthy development. To realize this potential, however, they needed to develop in a suitable environment, a diverse community with adequate physical and social resources. The initially enrolled families lived in a dull and restricted environment, with few physical and intellectual resources. In order for them to be healthier, their environment had to give them more choices and tools. These sponsors felt that health would develop only "within a society sufficiently mixed and varied to provide for the needs of mind and spirit as well as of the body" (p. 6). To meet this goal, they designed a new Pioneer Health Center.

The new center had to be large enough to accommodate at least 2000 people. It was to be based on the family unit, but it would deal with problems of family ill health by intervening at the next higher level of social organization—that is, by providing a more healthy social community, whose members and resources could encourage healthy behavior and healthy attitudes among one another. The core of the program would be around major points in the family life cycle: pregnancy, childbirth, infant care, child development, and parental needs. From this, the staff could then provide attention to the growing youngsters and adolescents, and meet the needs of the adults, as they too moved through life's stages.

The new center would follow five principles:

- Its unit had to be the family, in its biological setting.
- Families had to be free to act as they would.
- The environment had to be diverse, so that there were adequate opportunities for choice.
- The total group had to be sufficiently large.
- The project's scientists had to be able to observe the families in their natural behavior.

The new center opened in 1935. It was a bold glass-enclosed building, whose three cantilevered concrete platforms were built around an enclosed central rectangular swimming pool. The ground floor consisted of a gymnasium, a theater, an outside space for skating, cycling, and other children's games, and an infants' nursery. There was also a beginners' swimming pool. The main floor contained the body of the pool. This was surrounded on one side by a cafeteria and on the other by a large hall which could be used for social occasions. The floor also housed the upper portions of the gym and theater. The second floor, like the first, was completely open, except for a small consultation area. The rest of the space was devoted to a library, a work-room, and large open areas for games or quiet activity.

The entire area was open and airy. People's activities could be observed from almost any place of view. The founders of the project designed their living space for this purpose:

> The whole building is in fact characterised by a design which invites social contact, allowing equally for the chance meeting, for formal and festive occasions as well as for quiet familiar grouping. It is a field for

acquaintanceship and for the development of friendships, and for the entertainment by the family of visiting friends and relations. In these times of disintegrated social and family life in our villages, towns, and still worse in cities, there is no longer any place like this. Nevertheless, man has a long history of such spaces that have met the needs of his social life and the tentative adventure of his children as they grew up: —the church, the forum, the market-place, the village green, the courtyard; comfortable protected spaces where every form of fruitful social activity could lodge itself (p. 69).

People came to the building for a number of social occasions. In this, it was like the 1930s British equivalent to a YMCA. There was swimming all the time, and groups clustered talking around the pool. People came in the late morning for lunch, in the late afternoon for tea, and later on for dinner. Mothers brought their children for day care, then attended classes themselves in nutrition or child care, or simply read in the library. Teenagers socialized after school and held dances on the weekends. Men can by to socialize and have a beer before dinnertime. Many families were drawn in by their teenage children, who were eager to make use of the building's resources.

They would come and ask how they could become members. All they had to do was pay a small weekly sum and undergo a periodic health overhaul. Then they could use the facilities as often as they wished.

The Peckham Center was quite unlike a medical clinic. The physicians in attendance hated the term *doctor*—they called themselves "biologists" instead—and they did not provide routine medical care. Mainly they observed the interactions among families and individuals. Their medical/biological intervention was focused upon pregnancy and child care issues and issues of daily family life, and they were not a substitute for the local dispensary. Nor did the "staff" provide the service for the "patients." Indeed, Peckham operated on a principle of self-service. Older members were supposed to help orient the newer ones. Swimmers were supposed to help teach the nonswimmers. People were encouraged to share what they knew, what they were interested in, what they'd learned through their work, through reading and hobbies. People were on an informal basis with one another, and the atmosphere allowed for people's difference, and showed a concern for the needs and rhythms of people's lives.

Families, on first joining, were given an "enrollment talk." This was a general orientation on a day all family members could be present, often Saturday. The "biologists" explained the center's focus on health and outlined the purpose of the yearly health overhaul. They made their own interests clear; they wanted to study health and find out the ways by which it could best be achieved. Once this was presented, the family could choose to join. The founders' writings about Peckham emphasized its concern with the social development of its families. Pearse and Crocker talk about the "social starvation" of young families, and their need for greater contact with others. Their anecdotal accounts show the transformation of shy hitherto-housebound wives afraid of social contact outside the home to warm and outgoing women with friends in the club and an enriched married life. They talk about the overweight matron afraid of the swimming pool who gradually begins to exercise, and who moves from that act of involvement in the broader community to other such interaction. They talk about the social development of teenagers, and describe glowingly the rich social atmosphere that could be observed in the Peckham Center on any evening or weekend: youths forming friendships, young couples going to dances, people listening to others in the "club" talking about their lives and experiences, people dropping by for a cup of tea or a glass of beer and some time with friends. A variety of activities, from Ping-Pong to sewing, trampoline to drawing, darts to fencing, were all offered to the enrolled family members.

The yearly health overhaul was not to be confused with a medical evaluation or checkup. Its purpose was not the discovery of sickness. Rather it was for appraising the level of family health—the physical efficiency of the family and its members, and their capacity for individual, family, and social activity. The health overhaul included laboratory tests, physical examinations of all family members, and a family consultation in which each member was addressed and evaluated in turn, and in which the health of the whole family was then discussed. The idea was remarkably bold and innovative for its time, a fact which is proved by the paucity of imitators even to this day. The staff members' other activities seemed mainly in the area of health education and counseling. Psychotherapists were not part of the group. In fact, it would seem that the Peckham "biologists" did not share a view of illness dwelling in the psyche apart from the family and social context, and they had no use for psychology. Instead, they offered sex education for teenagers, premarital consultations, immunizations against infectious diseases, ante- and postnatal care (but not deliveries), infant care, contraceptive advice, and so on. They were always available, however, for consultation with members of the center, if the latter was concerned with any family or other problem.

The further findings of the Peckham Experiment are beyond the scope of this book. It should be pointed out that the project was never financially autonomous, but always relied on the support of sympathetic benefactors. Yet this experience represents a milestone in the history of attempts to view health from the broadest of all perspectives, and to provide family-oriented *health* care in a social, community-oriented setting. Although the Peckham Experiment itself has mainly ended, it still finds imitators across the world, and the writings of its "biologist" founders continue to be studied with fascination to this day.

FIVE

What's Been Tried: 1945 to the Present

Efforts to provide collaborative care have appeared in clusters—in the years around 1945, again in the early 1960s, and again in the early 1970s. This chapter looks at some of these recent antecedents, beginning with an examination of the contribution of social work to the field.

CONTRIBUTIONS FROM SOCIAL WORK

For generations, attention to psychosocial dimensions of health problems has been understood as a special domain for social work. One of the best places to find answers about the collaborative process, then, is the history of this field's involvement in health care.

Nineteenth century public health programs had brought different professionals together, uniting their efforts through a common commitment to the health of poor and disadvantaged, often immigrant, people. As medicine became more and more successful, however, and more and more specialized, its own purlieu became narrower; and physicians' desire to work alongside other professionals lost steam. At the same time, physicians seemed to lose interest in the social dimensions of health care. This territory became ceded to the social workers—both those attached to medical programs and those independent of medical programs—who appeared eager to take this area for their own province anyway. Indeed, social workers early on became experts in the team approach to health care, and they have written and contributed more to the topic than any other discipline.

Social work's involvement in health care thus began in the last third of the nineteenth century, and its broad societal orientation taught the relation of health and illness to coeval social and environmental factors. Social work grew up in close association with the halfway houses, ethnic-based clinics, milk depots, maternity and child health centers, and burgeoning community health clinics. The acknowledged date of its entry into collaborative health care activity, however, is 1905, when Dr. Richard Cabot of the Massachusetts General Hospital invited social workers into that facility, because he understood that family issues, housing conditions, and work factors were all involved in the illnesses being treated in the hospital's clinics. Since then, social workers have been an integral part of collaborative care in tertiary settings, have linked their teaching and training programs with those of other large health care institutions, and have carved out specific role responsibilities in such areas as chronic illness, disability, mental health, and public health. This work has provided the material basis for, and their systemic process-oriented outlook has provided the overall perspective for a penetrating critique of collaborative work in the health care field.

The tradition of medical social work made social work a bastion for the view that people's health problems were related to their social conditions, such as poverty, lack of skills, aging, poor housing conditions, and unemployment. Medical social workers became associated with large voluntary health organizations, community health centers, and the big urban hospitals, especially those in the northeast and midwest where the profession and its ideology most strongly developed. Medical social work was linked to the developing social welfare agencies as well. (For an extensive history of medical social work, compare Bracht, 1978; Kerson, 1982; Huntington, 1981; Miller and Rehr, 1983; and Estes, 1984; as well as the journal *Social Work in Health Care*.)

Private Practice Settings

Until recently, however, social workers worked mainly in tertiary care settings or in various social work agencies, and tended not to work in private practice settings, either on their own or with primary care physicians. They had participated, though, in a number of innovative projects, especially in New York City, which used different disciplines in providing comprehensive health care. I am thinking here of work at Montefiore Hospital (Levenson, 1984) and the Josiah Macy-sponsored project which was written up by H.B. Richardson as *Patients Have Families* (1948).

In the 1960s, both in the United States and elsewhere, the idea of a team approach to health care flourished once again. Linked to the community health movement in the United States and to the maturation of general practice abroad, it rested on a sound basis in fact: physicians simply had no time to see the number of people who sought their help for mainly emotional problems. In addition, people were questioning that the physician was even the correct practitioner to provide such care.

The notion that physicians alone cannot provide comprehensive health care is not new. The general estimate is that between 20 and 50 percent of patients coming to a physician have pressing psychosocial concerns. Physicians, however, usually lack both the time and the training to deal adequately with all these problems, although most GPs or FPs do in fact cope with a large number of their patients' psychosocial ills. Because of these limitations, "an important gap in domiciliary medical care, neglect of which leads to a continuing quantum of illness and unhappiness" (Forman and Fairbairn, 1968, p. 5), practitioners have been exploring team approaches to health care for decades. Scattered innovative moves to bring social workers into practice settings took place in the Netherlands, Great Britain, Israel, and the United States. The Institute of Social Medicine at Nijmegen University used social work-physician teams to study the social sources and social settings of illness. Social workers were assigned to work with patients from three general practices (Mertens, cited by Forman and Fairbairn, 1968, p. 4).

In England, a number of demonstration projects had their beginnings in the work of Professor Richard Scott and the social worker Jane Paterson, who worked together at the Edinburgh University General Practice Teaching Unit for 20 years. In the 1950s Backett, Maybin and Dudgeon (1957) investigated the social work content of a Northern Irish practice over a one year period and concluded that 12 percent of the families in the practice needed social work help. They proposed that a specially trained social worker could handle the work of a practice of 4000 patients. Other work was carried out by Dongray in Manchester (1958, 1962) and by Collins, who was attached to a Cardiff group medical practice for a year (1965).

As Goldberg and Neill (1972, p. 19) note:

Teamwork between doctors, social workers and other specialists was to
be the cornerstone of the health centres envisaged in the National Health
Services Act of 1947, but . . . this idea did not catch on among general
practitioners, and hardly any health centres came into being in the fif-
ties. The few which did . . . did not function with integrated teams, but
merely provided common premises in which general practitioners, health
visitors, infant welfare and child guidance clinics were located.

As general practitioners began to realize the practical advantages
of forming group practices, thereby pooling their resources, conditions developed that made it feasible for them to employ ancillary
staff. Of course, employing a social worker rested on the physicians'
conviction that social factors were important to their patients' health.
By 1965 the notion of local health centers, staffed by multidisciplinary teams, had gained some strength in Great Britain, just as it had in
the United States at the same time. Richard Scott (1965, cited in Goldberg and Neill, pp. 17-18) provided a brief for this position, arguing
that:

the aetiology of much of the disease we encounter in general practice,
and many of the factors which complicate our management of the sick
person, have their origins in social maladjustment and in inadequate or
faulty interpersonal relationships. To the extent that this is so our therapy will become less concerned with manipulating the patient's blood
chemistry and more preoccupied with the physical, economic and social
factors in the patient's environment. The decision which is taken as to
whether such problems will be regarded as the sole responsibility of the
medical profession or . . . as a field which requires a full partnership between medicine and other related social agencies, will be a major factor
in determining the future of general practice.

Scott urged that a social worker be brought into the general practice team. The ensuing ten years saw a number of projects in Great
Britain that investigated exactly this—adding a social worker to an
on-going (often group) medical practice.

Forman and Fairbairn's book *Social Casework in General Practice*
(1968) is one of the first descriptions of this kind of experience. Although written almost 20 years ago, its observations are as fresh and
relevant to work today as if they were written last week, and they
touch on almost every conceivable area involved in the process of integrating a social worker (or other "psychosocially-oriented figure")
into a family medical practice.

The authors report the three-year experience of adding a social
worker to a six-physician group medical practice. The project was

underwritten by a philanthropic grant. Its main object was to estimate the value of attaching a medical social worker to a group medical practice; but it also sought to analyze the type of problems referred to her, to estimate the need for such psychosocial work in the practice, and to estimate the value of such a site in helping a medical social worker contact those in need of her services.

The practice was a country town of 20,000 people, evenly divided between town and rural life. Many families had been in the practice for generations, and there were widespread family-to-practice loyalties.

One of the marvels of this book is that it is written in two parts. The first describes the experience from the physician's point of view; the second, from the social worker's perspective.

The physician concludes that adding an almoner was valuable because of the casework (therapy) services she provided and because of her ability in mobilizing the available social resources. He feels that direct patient referral from the GP to the social worker is a sound practice, preferable to the social worker's screening or sampling the practice in a random way. He has no doubt that adding such a figure improved the quality of care, especially in areas in which care had previously been weak. Furthermore, patients are felt to be quite accepting of the social worker.

The physician then describes the "Patient-GP-Medical Social Worker triangle," and discusses how the collaborating professionals gradually learned to communicate ideas and insights to one another. (I couldn't help thinking that Mac Baird and Bill Doherty were sitting in the room as this section was being written. Certainly they [and most of us] would have found Forman and Fairbairn to be kindred spirits.) The addition of a social worker improves communication within the practice, both between physician and patient and between the physicians and their social worker colleague. At the same time, the physician feels it important that the social worker maintain her own independence.

Of the 409 cases referred to the social worker, the GPs rate her contribution as helpful in 93 percent. They feel her main contribution lies in providing therapy (59%) and in establishing links with social service agencies (62%). Of the total group of referred patients, almost all (99%) are felt to have had problems with social "circumstances," such as housing, schooling, occupation, finance, and aging, as well as life-stage personal problems. In only half of the referrals is physical illness estimated to be a contributing factor to the difficulty. Half the patients are felt to have had substantial personality difficulties as part of the presenting problem. The physicians feel the almoner saved them time, and did work that would otherwise not have been done by anyone else in the office. They also feel that a general practice is an excellent site for a medical social worker: access to patients needing their services is simplified, the physician's load is eased, the patients are accepting, continuity of care is a positive factor, and the social worker can preserve her independence.

The social worker's part of the book focuses as much on the process of her involvement as on its results. For example, she points out that her joining the practice had a definite impact on how the physicians thought: their referring behavior changed as they learned what she could do.

She feels her main contribution lay in the *assessment* of the problems encountered. The patients felt most likely to benefit from medicosocial help include (1) those who repeatedly come to the GP with symptoms but have no demonstrable disease: their problem is felt due mainly to social difficulties; (2) socially inadequate patients, whose problems are due to lack of money, lack of adequate housing, and so on, "with a troop of children who are prey to every passing infection"; (3) those who remain unwell after a physical illness; and (4) families with a continuing burden of chronic disablement. Her response to these referrals includes casework dealing with the complex social and emotional situations (therapy), and evaluation and referral to appropriate social service agencies. In addition, the social worker agrees that her presence and perspective increased the physicians' awareness of the social factors in their patients' lives, and she modestly speculates on the role of a social worker in educating GPs about these issues.

One wonders why only 100 patients a year were referred to the almoner out of a practice of 14,400 (and even this was felt to represent a large caseload for her). If the percentage referred were closer to the figure in our own and other practices—about 15 to 20 percent of patients are felt to have significant emotional/social problems, and of these about one-quarter are referred for treatment—then that would mean that 4 to 5 percent of the practice, not 1 percent, would be seen by the social worker. This seems to me to represent an even greater need for such collaborative care.

Goldberg and Neill (1972), following in the tradition of the previous authors, pursued a similar project in Caversham. In this undertaking, also funded by private philanthropic efforts, a social worker joined a four-physician group medical practice in a London borough for a five-year period. The practice is described as very open and community-based, with 9000 patients, 1000 of whom were eventually referred to the social worker. Many more patients were discussed without being officially referred.

Goldberg and Neill painstakingly analyze the many factors involved in their work. Their data is extensive and very interesting for comparison's sake for anyone currently doing the same kind of work. At the beginning, the authors describe how a team approach affects physicians customarily used to the "possessive," "exclusive" interpersonal relationship between patient and physician. What happens when someone else is introduced into this dyad? Furthermore, what does the social worker bring to the relationship? Also, as it turns out, in spite of all the talk about collaborative care, most GPs in Great Britain seem very unfamiliar with what social workers know and can do. The authors conclude that GPs need to learn what social workers can provide.

Their book presents an excellent analysis of the specifics of the practice—the personnel, the physical setting, the referral process, the social worker's role. Its entire next section is devoted to "the caseload": the social worker's clients are analyzed category by category, and their problems and the social worker's responses are laid forth. Twice as many women as men were referred. Over a third were elderly; and two-thirds were either single, widowed, divorced, or separated. A third lived by themselves. Most of the referred patients had complained to their physician either of vague psychosomatic problems, emotional ill-health, or overt social problems; only two-fifths had presented their physician with definite physical complaints. Most patients, however, turned out to have a number of interrelated problems—for example, many patients with physical illness needed the provision of ancillary services (home care, Meals on Wheels) as well as emotional support. Hidden problems often emerged. Nearly a third of the patients spoke about family difficulties in their first interview. Nearly a quarter were worried about their health or were going through some personal crisis.

Evaluation of the patients' "main problems" was that a third were related to difficulties in family relationships, a fifth connected to material and environmental needs, and another fifth to worries about personal health or involvement in a personal crisis. Other categories were psychiatric difficulties and school or work problems.

A section entitled "social work in action" describes what the social worker did and is the most intriguing section of the book; it is dotted here and there with brief case histories. The simplest form of treatment consisted of providing clarification, assessment, advice, and information. This was given to 24 percent of the group referred. Twenty-eight percent were referred to other, outside social agencies.

The main form of treatment was what we might call short-term therapy. The social worker took on 43 percent of referred patients for this kind of casework treatment, most of which lasted less than three months, less than ten visits. Such short-term help appeared useful in a number of categories—people dealing with cross-cultural problems; people facing family problems, especially when loyalties are being split or when there is family separation; people in crisis; people facing terminal illness, death, and bereavement; people dealing with "accumulated stress and trigger events."

In addition to this short-term help, longer treatment was offered to some families that tended to fall into the "high-user" category and were felt to have many physical and mental handicaps.

Recommending their model to others, Goldberg and Neill argue that a social worker adds much to the general practice. The social worker's insights contribute to a more comprehensive diagnosis. She can more effectively link the practice to available community resources, and she brings a wide range of useful skills to her therapy and casework with patients and their families. Finally, the presence of a social worker in the practice stimulates mutual education between physician and social worker. In all of this, they feel, her contribution is greatest if she is seen as an equal partner with her medical and nonmedical colleagues.

In a similar recent paper, Justin and Shanks (1983) describe a collaborative effort between a family physician and a social worker in private practice in the midwestern United States. They found that social work counseling was helpful to the great majority of patients, and especially to the elderly. The most frequent reasons for referral were environmental problems (38%), emotional problems (25%), physical problems (22%), and family problems (15%). Referral to another agency was carried out in 62 percent of the cases, supportive casework in 19 percent, and providing necessary information in another 19 percent.

Many other reports have since appeared in the social work literature, not only advocating but also critiquing the collaborative process (compare Chapter 9). Social workers have analyzed collaboration with physicians, nurses, and others, and have examined the teamwork process in great detail. In the past 20 years, social workers have worked in community-based health programs, in tertiary-care hospitals, and, increasingly, in the private sector.

Current Social Work Involvement in Health Care

What is the current social worker involvement in health care? Approximately 60,000 of the 150,000 professionally qualified social workers currently work in the health care field. About two-thirds of them provide some form of mental health services. Most of the rest work in acute and long-term medical care facilities. A growing number, however, are joining with private medical practices to work with their patients' psychosocial needs, or are becoming involved in at least part-time private counseling.

Estes (1984, p. 4) provides a good summary of contemporary social work activity in health care. He lists five different functions social workers perform:

- Participate actively in all aspects of clinical case assessment, planning, treatment, service management, and patient follow up;
- Function as specialists in the psycho-social aspects of health care;
- Serve as consultants to practitioners of other health disciplines in helping to better understand and impact more effectively upon the complex psycho-social factors that directly affect patient care;
- Link patients and their families to the full spectrum of in-patient, out-patient and community-based health services;
- Facilitate patient and family access to the even greater array of health-related services available to them from literally thousands of human service agencies located communities all across the United States.

In addition to this, Estes notes, social workers also "function as health educators, patient advocates and ombudsmen," and as providers of primary health services.

The recent writings of Gilbert Greene focus even more sharply on the venues open to social workers in family medical practice. Promoting the idea of "family practice social work," Greene, Kruse and Arthurs (1985) have outlined the essentials for social workers in this new subspecialty. Another article by Greene and Kruse (unpublished manuscript) examines the openness of family physicians towards this kind of cooperation. As more and more efforts at collaboration occur, writings on the topic can be expected to increase.

OTHER COLLABORATIVE EFFORTS

Many other collaborative efforts have sprung up over the past several decades. These include a number of projects that took place in the 1940s and a wide outpouring of such programs that began in the 1960s and continued into the late 1970s.

In 1942 the psychiatrist Maurice Levine published *Psychotherapy in Medical Practice* (1942). Aimed at an audience of general practitioners, it purports to instruct them in basic forms of psychotherapy that could aid them in their practices. Chapters include "Methods [of Psychotherapy] for the General Practitioner," "Advanced Methods for the General Practitioner," "The Study of Psychogenic Factors," "The Problems of Parents and Children," and "Normality and Maturity." Levine felt that GPs, who admittedly saw "the majority of the psychologic problems in the community [p. vii]," could benefit from colleagial advice and treat such problems more efficiently. One of his guiding perspectives was to try and treat the "patient as a whole [p. xii]." Although Levine did not work with groups of GPs like, for example, Michael Balint in England, his interest in helping family physicians treat the patients who presented with psychological problems reflected a growing (albeit modest) trend toward the working together of psychosocially and medically oriented caregivers.

Between 1938 and 1943, the Josiah Macy, Jr. Foundation funded a critical project in interdisciplinary family-oriented care in New York City, the Study of the Family in Sickness and Health Care. The project's results are summarized by its director, H.B. Richardson in his book *Patients Have Families* (1948). This study brought together members of the Departments of Public Health, Medicine, and Psychiatry at Cornell University Medical College in an effort to examine the relationship between illness and people's family situation. Its staff also included social work and nursing professionals from New York Hospital. Utilizing a strong family perspective, these investigators studied 15 families intensively over a two-year period. Although theirs was essentially a small study project, they emerged with notions about the relationships between illness and the family that were decades ahead of their time. More than their findings, the researchers' perspective set the tone for an all-sided and contextual investigation of usually unchallenged concepts such as the "patient" and "diagnosis."

Richardson (1948) used the term *system* in its contemporary sense, applied to the understanding of health in a family context:

One of the effects of these underlying tendencies . . . is to set up a special sort of relationship between two individuals, which I shall call a reciprocating system. This is a simplified way of looking at one aspect of a family situation which may be highly complex. Characteristically the people involved tend to react on one another in a predictable manner with specified results. These systems also tend to perpetuate themselves, whether for better or for worse (p. 91).

It also was one of the first books to proclaim that:

The idea of disease as an entity which is limited to one person and can be transmitted to another, fades into the background, and disease becomes an integral part of the continuous process of living. The family is the unit of illness, because it is the unit of living (p. 76).

One chapter in the book deals with the cooperation between family physicians and their psychotherapy consultants. Other chapters explore additional aspects of collaborative care, such as the different perspectives the physician, nurse, and social worker bring to the care of the family. Throughout, Richardson's is an expanded view of the doctor-patient-family relationship, as is clear from his preface:

The profession of medicine progressed from the diseased organ to the total personality of the patient, and is now ready for the concept of the individual as a member of the family in its community setting. Coincident with this development a reverse process has been started in the community, to illness, to the individual personality. . . . The time is now as the physician thinks of a patient. They consider medicine as only one aspect of family welfare, and proceed in reverse, from the family in the community, to illness, to the individual personality. . . . The time is now ripe for a coordinated attack on the problems of family adjustment in relation to the maintenance of health and the treatment of illness (1948, p. xviii).

The first part of Richardson's book looks at "The Family as the Unit of Illness." It views the family in different contexts—hospital, community, home—and from different family members' viewpoints. It even sets out to develop a rudimentary (but highly sophisticated) typology of families, and introduces the notion of family equilibrium and family homeostasis, as well as the notion of the family as a system. The second part of the book moves to consider "The Family as the Unit of Treatment." This section looks at the role of the family practitioner, at the cooperation between family physician and psychiatrist, and at the roles of the medical social worker, the case worker, and the public health nurse in the treatment team.

More material about this program can be gleaned from Ransom's writings (1984), showing the links between the Macy-sponsored project and the developing systemic theories of Margaret Mead and Gregory Bateson. Richardson himself cites the inspiration of the earlier Peckham Experiment as a strong influence guiding the group's work.

The end of the Macy Foundation Study in New York dovetailed with the development of the HIP—an early prepaid group HMO—as well as with the concomitant rise of the Kaiser-Permanente prepaid family health program in California. In New York, led by Dr. George A. Silver, the Family Health Maintenance Demonstration project at Montefiore took up where Richardson's project had left off. Utilizing a team approach to the provision of health care, the Montefiore project operated for a decade throughout the 1950s, pioneering many community-oriented approaches to family health and learning by firsthand experience the tribulations of the health care team.

Silver's conceptualization of this project combined his keen sense of the changing medical scene with an appreciation of the interrelationship between physical and emotional factors in health and disease and an earnest desire to focus on preventive medicine from a community/ecology perspective:

> Four major developments gave impetus to the idea of Family Health Maintenance. . . . First . . . was the recognition of the importance of prevention in disease and professional dedication to the concept of prevention. Second was the changing nature of medical practice deriving from the fact that chronic illness and psychiatric problems with their implications increased in relative importance. Third was the growing conviction that mental and physical health were interrelated and that emotions had some part to play in disease causation and maintenance. Fourth was the changing role of professional workers in the medical field, as a result of altered technology; the clashing expectations of patient and doctor; and the growing importance of paramedical workers (Silver, 1974, p. 3).

Silver cites both the Peckham Experiment and Sidney Kark's work in South Africa as precursors of his own program. Building on the work of these predecessors, the Montefiore program utilized regular family health conferences and insisted (in theory) on taking the family as both the living unit and the unit of treatment. Many of its innovations served to encourage later community-based projects in the

1960s, especially those in underserved, poor and minority communities. Silver's work was finally written up as *Family Medical Care: A Design for Health Maintenance* in 1974.

The Montefiore work was filled with reformist zeal. Silver saw medical care as being at a crisis point. He believed that providers had to organize in teams to meet the full panoply of patients' needs; and that these teams should center in the community, not in the hospital. He held that families should be evaluated in their own right, not by some preconceived notion; and he was curiously attracted to the notion that "harmony" in living was somehow linked to family health (p. 29), a view that anticipated Antonovsky's writings on the subject (1979).

The Montefiore project combined study of family health and illness with the actual, interdisciplinary provision of medical care. It focused on health promotion and especially on meeting the needs of the family's children. The interdisciplinary teams—physician, nurse, social worker—cared for over 120 families over a five-year period. Their data from this group was then compared with a control sample of HIP members.

Although the project's results seemed favorable—more of its patients were satisfied with their health care than were control families; health status seemed improved compared to the control group; half as many study families left the HIP as control families—there were also a number of problems. Not the least of these involved intra-team disputes and wranglings over role, responsibility, authority, and turf. Team members held different assumptions and different priorities, and coordination proved easier in word than in deed.

"The Demonstration," as it was called, came up with some provocative findings. For example, there was a high degree of emotional difficulty in presumably normal families, which Silver speculates is due to some self-healing or coping factor that enabled them to compensate without asking for outside aid. The group found that frequent routine health examinations were not very productive, and instead proposed that a routine team conference on health problems be held in their place. Most interesting were the views about staff dispute and role difficulty. If one reads between the lines, there appeared to be much difficulty integrating the social worker with the more medical team members. Attitudes seemed hard to break down, and cultural, class and social influences loomed as critical factors in the success of team-provided health care.

One problem with the Demonstration was its inability to move beyond the different component disciplines. Cooperation seemed hard to obtain. Members of the teams actually worked apart from one another, and there was little time for sharing information and working out a common assessment or treatment program. Nor did the family really seem to be the focus of care. In spite of the rhetoric, Silver downplayed the notion of any resurgence of the family physician—even in 1974 when the second edition of his book came out!—and focused on care provided by internists. The shadow of the Montefiore medical empire (that is, specialist care) hung over the Demonstration. Nor was Silver drawn to the systemic, communicative/understandable nature of family interaction, but rather seemed more centered on the basic needs of the families in his project. The most systemic aspect of his work actually strikes me as the understanding of interprofessional rivalry, which, if I am not mistaken, was a contribution Eliot Freidson, the medical sociologist, made in working with the project as a consultant.

Summing up the project's difficulties, Ransom (1985, p. 375) comments:

> On the one hand, the Demonstration's central purpose, the delivery of comprehensive family-focussed health care, never gave itself a chance. . . . There were many reasons why: its location in a subspecialty-dominated academic medical environment, its reliance as "family doctors" on internists whose concern was with "everything that goes on inside the skin," its unwieldy teams whose members did not share a common approach . . . and its failure to borrow or construct a social-interactional model of the family as a dynamic system. In short, it was the lack of a necessary imagination . . . that kept them from achieving their most innovative ambition.

THE 1960S

The work at Montefiore served as a source of great encouragement to those who wanted to take medical care more broadly into the community. In the 1960s all of society seemed to be experiencing a sense of change, and many innovative projects took shape, often qualifying for government backing at a time when the Great Society was enacting the reform programs of Medicaid, Medicare, and community health centers. Funds were available for a number of community-based projects, and many health professionals appeared willing to work in such projects in hopes of bettering the health care system, especially in poor and minority communities. The community health center movement thus developed with great enthusiasm at places such as Montefiore (Wise, 1972; Wise et al., 1974) and Gouverneur Hospitals in New York City (compare Auerswald [1983], Cook County Hospital in Chicago, Lincoln Hospital in the Bronx, and "free clinics" in many places). Many of these programs used a team concept. Usually, however, the teams were biomedically oriented; they did not, as a rule, focus on the psychosocial factors that affected people's health so much as on the socioeconomic ones that did. (One important exception was the work in New Haven [see Coleman, 1979], which did join mental health professionals to community primary care.) Usually, however, the orientation encouraged looking externally for the main source of people's unhappiness; there was in fact a general mistrust of social workers (who worked for the welfare department, not for the patient/client), therapists (who cooled out the potential for struggle latent in the community), and psychoanalytic language (which appeared to make people responsible for their own suffering).

The health activists of the 1970s formed interdisciplinary organizations such as the Medical Committee for Human Rights (MCHR), which united professionals from different fields in working for the same radical, humanitarian, and antiwar causes. The Women's Movement, the Black Liberation struggle, the Civil Rights Movement, and the anti-Vietnam War Movement, all of which were simultaneously happening, stretched people's sense of how much needed to be done to move society towards its highest potential. Community health centers were sites of intense political and professional work where much was tried, and much was learned.

The community health center movement developed in many places at once—New York, Oakland, Seattle, Boston, Chicago, New Haven. Wherever the movement was, health care activity could be found. Health collectives sprung up, especially around women's health issues (compare the "Our Bodies, Our Selves" group in Boston and women's health clinics in almost every major city). Mainstream health institutions were affected by the changes in outlook taking place among their staff and students. Hospitals such as Montefiore and Gouverneur in New York City, Cook County in Chicago, and Lincoln in the Bronx became organizing centers.

From this enthusiasm, a multitude of collaborative efforts burst forth, which involved thousands of health care workers and operated for at least a decade. Today, however, these experiences remain widely ignored. Many of the programs collapsed suddenly, when their funds were stopped in the late 1970s, and few programs summed up their work. Instead, we are left with many statements from the beginning of these groups, exhortations to the team concept and team care, but little overall evaluation of what happened, what went wrong, what was good, and what was bad.

One such program was the Valentine Lane Family Practice connected with the Montefiore Hospital in the Bronx. The following description of this program is taken from an interview with Rita Ulrich, M.S.W. (1985, p. 88), who served as the social worker-family consultant in the practice:

> Valentine Lane was a family- and community-oriented primary health care practice, affiliated with Montefiore Hospital in the Bronx. It had a staff of four practitioners . . . a family nurse practitioner . . . an internist . . . a pediatrician . . . and me. . . . We were hired in June, 1974, by the Institute for Health Team Development to become a collaborative health care team. We were supposed to become a "model team," providing health care services, as well as teaching other health professionals about interdisciplinary collaboration. . . . These teams were needed to provide comprehensive health care, because no one provider could do it all alone. But [then] it seemed that professional training was actually working *against* collaboration: By the time we became professionals in our various disciplines, collaboration was almost impossible without a very specific intervention to help it along.

Because of this, the Robert Wood Johnson Foundation funded interdisciplinary programs at five major university centers, involving the faculties of medicine, nursing, social work, dentistry, and pharmacy. It then set about to train the faculty of this program, by creating model teams such as Valentine Lane. The team spent a concentrated period of time focusing on its own process and making its plans; then it began its work.

From the start there was a conflict between the task of being a model team for the Foundation and the task of providing services to its patients and their community. Beyond this, though, there was a conflict between the project's relying on Foundation dollars for its budget and its acknowledged purpose of showing that such a collaborative team could turn a profit in private practice. Rita Ulrich (1985, pp. 91-92) says:

> The project was supposed to develop a replicable model for fee-for-service, that is, private practice. But we were in no way "private practice. . . ." We were fee-for-service. But we were part of a major teaching insti-

tution and a major hospital center, and we were on salary from them. We . . . had constraints on us that private practice never had. . . . Most of all, we didn't have to be as accountable from a cost effective standpoint. . . . That's why we eventually went under. We were supposed to cover our costs, but as it wound up we didn't pay enough attention to it. . . . We didn't realize the importance of being cost-effective until it was too late. We relied on outside funding.

When funding was eventually stopped, Valentine Lane, as it had existed, had to end. Never having seriously addressed the question of managing on its own, it was ill-prepared to revise its staff's schedules, argue with the Medicaid structure which reimbursed them at private practice rates even though it had the bureaucratic structure of a hospital clinic. It could not meet its own budget and folded.

In her interview, Ulrich (1985) comments further on the notion of cost-effectiveness:

Another part of the problem was that the criteria for cost-effectiveness were based on the traditional medical model, which was that you make an intervention and then you have a measureable outcome. But we were talking about making interventions, family interventions, whose outcome you might not be able to measure for years. For instance, one of our early families was chaotic and dysfunctional. The father was hospitalized on the average of once every two months. He was being treated for serious heart disease. We all worked very closely with this family. It soon became apparent that he was hyperventilating. I mean, it seems ridiculously simple now, but it wasn't then. And with some considerable team effort, the problem was reframed from being a heart condition to being a condition which was much less serious, although still disabling. The patient and his family were helped to function a little better. It saved the health care system an enormous amount of money, saved the family an enormous amount of pain and anguish. We worked with the wife. We worked with the kids. This was the kind of thing we did. However, that could take years. It was not something you could "measure an outcome of" in six or eight months in the traditional way. But we were not smart enough, not experienced enough, to set up an evaluation component that *could* measure what we did. That, ultimately, was a major factor in our downfall. We didn't know how to convert a medical study into a health care study that measured "functionalism" over an extended period of time (p. 92).

Saving money is hard, because initially you don't save money, you spend it. You only save in the long run, and that's what you need to demonstrate. You'll save money because people are not hospitalized as often. You'll save money because they're learning to manage and func-

tion better, using less costly resources, not going to mental health clinics
(p. 101).

Ulrich describes other aspects of Valentine Lane—the patients'
warm acceptance of the team approach, the community's enthusiasm
over the extent of services available, the project's innovative use of
patients as staff helping other patients. Although there were indeed
some personality conflicts among the staff, she feels this was not a
major factor in the project's demise. That was due, she feels, to economic factors. In looking back, she feels her experience with collaborative care was tremendously exciting and rewarding. But there were
lessons to be learned:

> People who band together to provide primary health care services need
> to look consciously at their interdependence. Collaboration is a learned
> skill, not intuitive behavior. It's critical for each member to define his
> or her professional uniqueness. They'd also have to be special kinds of
> people, today, with a commitment to a shared vision of what health
> care should be. Doing that feels like swimming upstream to me. But I
> do think it's a viable model (Ulrich, 1985, p. 101).

Similar kinds of experience happened to hundreds of health care
workers involved in collaborative, community-based attempts at providing health care in the 1970-1980 decade.

Other aspects of the "spirit of the 1960s" also deserve mention.
H. Jack Geiger and others worked to establish rural health clinics in
Mississippi, thus linking the Civil Rights Movement and the community health movement. Some groups utilized mobile crisis units, political health care teams, women's health collectives, and community-
based health clinics to carry health care to the people they served.
Teams often worked hard on community outreach and tried to de-
mystify medical secrets—activities that might today be reframed as
self-help and patient-education.

And yet, the 1960s community health care teams, interdisciplinary as they were, frequently stuck closely to the biomedical model.
Their personnel might include pediatricians, internists, nurse practitioners, and social workers, but they usually did not view counseling
as one of their central tasks. It seemed beyond the pale. The more
conventional personnel felt medical care should be more narrowly
focused around specific health care needs, such as preventing infant
mortality, identifying lead poisoning and sickle cell disease, and so

on. The more radical personnel looked toward the systemic levels of the community and state, not the family.

In a sense, this wing indeed held to a biopsychosocial perspective, but it tended to be political, concerned with the consequences of macrosystems on people's health. These people analyzed the effects of imperialism, racism, and sexism on health care, and tried to organize the community (such as it was) to struggle against these injustices in the larger system. To them, therapy was part of the problem, not part of the solution. In addition, the family was not the sacred entity it has become today, but was an institution to be mistrusted. People with a narrower perspective thus avoided contextual issues, and people with a broader perspective mistrusted counseling and worked for larger-scale change instead.

Not only do the lessons of the 1960s still need to be written down and analyzed, so too do the lessons of the decade which followed, for in the 1970s a number of collaborative efforts in health care were attempted. (A newly published work, *Mental Health Practices in Primary Care Settings: An Annotated Bibliography 1977-85*, edited by Greg Wilkinson [New York, Tavistock, 1985], gathers over 500 references of work which is—at least in some ways—collaborative. The interested reader is encouraged to peruse this volume to get a flavor of the intense amount of collaborative work that has been going on—consultation-liaison psychiatry, mental health services in primary care clinics, psychotherapeutic activity in general practice, primary care management of emotional disorders, questions of referral and so on.) The enthusiasm for conjoint work seemed infectious. Sadly, many of these efforts, even those that occurred a scant ten years ago, have not been popularized among those currently in training programs today (another example of the lack of a historical sense in the United States).

Today's context for health care differs in many ways from the 1960s and 1970s—for example, the rise of family medicine, the sophistication and maturity of family therapy, the doctor glut (not physician shortage), the concern with cutting costs rather than expanding services, the absence of any of the broad mass movements of the 1960s. Let us now turn to an examination of the current basis for collaborative health care and to the actual forms of such care that exist.

SIX

The Organization of Collaborative Health Care

The last widespread attempts at providing collaborative health care in the United States took place between 1965 and 1975. By the late 1970s most of these efforts had been abandoned; the foundations and agencies that had sponsored them, enthusiastically promoting the notion of the health care team, had by then concluded that collaborative care was no longer practicable. They withdrew their funds, and the programs, which had relied on them to meet their operating costs, collapsed.

What led these sponsors to decide that collaborative care could not work? Their reasons seem little related to the programs' actual results. Rather, the programs' sponsors changed their focus from developing interdisciplinary health care teams toward cutting the health care costs that had increased wildly in this period. It was now against the tide to advocate more rather than fewer providers. This policy coincided with a recognition of today's doctor glut as opposed to the previously well-publicized primary health care manpower shortage, and it has led to the downgrading of many physician extender programs as well (except in HMOs, where extenders—nurse practitioners and physician assistants—are seen as cheaper forms of medical manpower). The shift in policy also involved the resurgence of the more biomedical view of health care and a new get-tough policy towards the health care of the poor. The health care teams had engendered many problems, especially concerning communication, struggles over turf, and hierarchy. Abandoning them seemed simple and expedient.

The collaborative health care efforts of the 1970s were abandoned long before their results were in. Their results have never been fully summed up, nor their lessons been made available. Their long-term results were not available when these projects were terminated. (Might an extra $10 spent in the first five years of a program save $50 over the next five? How does one assess the health of a community—by its overall health care costs? by the types of illnesses it has? But what, if access to care is trimmed during the study period? Do you emphasize the actual savings of dollars or look at the types of illnesses in the community? How do you evaluate preventive work?)

As those programs collapsed, their staff scurried for other positions. Burnout and demoralization frequently kept people from looking back to reexamine what they had been doing for the previous four or five years. Projects often simply ended, with no attempt at summing-up.

To me, it seems inappropriate to apply conclusions reached in this context in 1975 to the medical scene of the late 1980s. The situation today differs markedly from what it was two decades ago. For example, family medicine did not exist in the 1960s, and was just beginning to develop by 1975. Family therapy, which did exist in 1965-1975, had not yet attained the breadth of scope it has achieved today. These groups are the twin bulwarks for collaborative health care in the 1980s and 1990s. Over the past 20 years, they have developed and matured and are now capable of working productively together to help develop a collaborative model of care.

THE BASIS FOR COLLABORATIVE CARE: FAMILY THERAPY/COUNSELING FIELDS AND PRIMARY CARE (FAMILY) MEDICINE

The people who provide the basis for collaborative health care practice come from the thousands of family (and other family-oriented primary care) physicians and family-oriented counselors and therapists. These two groups of health practitioners were in early stages of development in the 1960s, when the last attempts at collaborative health care occurred.

Family Medicine

As stated earlier, most Americans prefer having a family doctor. Family physicians have now "come back" and are available in most places to provide and coordinate family-oriented care.

Family medicine began as a protest against the fragmentation and dehumanization of American medicine. Its founders were idealists and dissidents—humanists, existentialists, and renegades—committed to caring for people in a family context rather than with perpetuating organ-system medicine. Many of them had been practicing physicians, not academics, but they were attracted to the new discipline by its model of care, which added psychosocial dimensions to the usual notions of health care. Today, the orientation of family practice still contrasts with that of specialist medical care, where physicians busily refer to one another, each one caring for a different member of the family, or a different organ system.

The term *family medicine* was taken almost by accident, it seems, but was then parlayed into a political asset. The field owed its growth to several factors: a desire to resuscitate the old-time family doctor, fanned by the old-time GPs as well as by patients' preference for a family physician; increased pressures by the government and the insurance industry to cut the costs of medical care by providing more generalists; an ideological concern with treating the "whole" patient in his or her family context—holistic health—as contrasted to the increasing fragmentation of medical services in the United States; as well as an appreciation on some physicians' parts of the deeper, psychosocial aspects of the doctor-patient relationship.

For a time, the field struggled. It acted on its family orientation by inviting professionals from the social and behavioral sciences into its burgeoning departments. From the start, social workers, psychologists, and others interested in family process and dynamics joined the field. Then, as time went on, family medicine became more and more successful; instead of looking to unite the renegades and eclectics, its leaders now looked to rejoin the mainstream of American medicine. The ensuing conflicts, beyond the scope of this book, have nonetheless affected the course and direction of all of medical practice.

The promise of family medicine can be drawn from the attitudes of its leaders. G. Gayle Stephens has written often about the moral responsibility of the family physician; he often cites existentialist theologians like Reinhold Niebuhr or Martin Buber. Lynn Carmichael (1983, pp. 126-127) has written that 80 percent of family practice follows the "relational model," which is:

> not concerned with cure or control of disease but rather with the attention, support, and comfort the patient receives. The physician acts on the basis of what ought to be done. . . . This model assumes action for

social and affectual and not instrumental purposes. Concern is with feelings, relationships, and the skills to cope with mental and physical stress. The doctor and the patient become participants in this action and process criteria such as style, manner, and responsiveness are used for evaluation.

As an organized discipline, family medicine is still immersed in controversy, and a gamut of opinions exists among its practitioners. In general, family physicians fall into two main groups: (1) Older general practitioners, still mainly practicing by themselves, who have not received residency training, but who kept the tradition of family practice live between the years 1940 to 1970. (2) Younger, mainly residency-trained family practitioners, including an increasing number of women, who tend to work in groups. Sharp disputes have emerged over the use of family therapy in family medicine and over the extent to which medicine should follow a biopsychosocial model.

Family practitioners can also be divided into two main ideological groupings: (1) The larger group, about 80 percent, appears eager to make family medicine similar to other medical fields. It emphasizes a biomedical approach to health and illness, and looks favorably toward family medicine's growing acceptance by the rest of organized medicine. (I call this the "tail of the dog" or "medical caboose" mentality.) (2) The smaller group includes many of the field's founders, as well as some younger residency-trained family practitioners. It rejects the biomedical model as too narrow, and instead advocates the "biopsychosocial" model of illness. Its adherents include physicians who consider themselves "systems thinkers." Some of them have also obtained training in the behavioral sciences or family therapy, and try to treat both the emotional and the physical aspects of their patients' difficulties.

The minority position challenges traditional medicine by providing a working model of how health care can integrate psychological insights and treatment into traditional medical care. It proposes an ideological alternative in medical practice today and its members constitute the potential family medicine component in collaborative health care practice.

Other Primary Medical Care Specialties

Over the past two or three decades, medicine has also seen the development of a primary care movement. This tendency arose in the late 1960s, spurred by reports that the number of specialists in American medicine was approaching 80 percent, and that this was a main factor in the ever-escalating costs of medical care. Arising as the community health center movement was fading, the primary care movement provided a new locus for funds for the traditional specialties of internal medicine, obstetrics-gynecology, and pediatrics. The movement trumpeted the need for more general physicians, but yet it seemed peculiarly fixated on the already existing departments of primary care specialties—in other words, on some parts of the already dominant medical establishment. The primary care movement did not address the need for more family physicians. Rather, it held that family physicians were a relic of the past. Representatives of the primary care fields consistently opposed the start-up of family medicine departments in their medical schools (Tufts, Boston University, Harvard, Columbia) and instead spoke about their own disciplines' abilities to provide primary care services.

The rhetoric of primary care medicine and family medicine overlapped on several counts, of course. Each wished to provide continuous and accessible as well as first-line care; each was willing to be a medical gatekeeper, cost-effectively referring patients to other (higher-priced) specialists only when "really" necessary. Differences had to do with their view of the family. Family physicians were eager to take on the provision of care from "cradle to grave," treating the elderly, the newborn, and everyone in between, in their family/dynamic context. The primary care fields limited their patients to a particular group: adults, women of child-bearing age, children. Yet, in spite of some elements of conflict, the primary care fields today are filled with many astute clinicians who have pursued a broad psychosocial approach for years. They have charted a tradition of comprehensive care from a primary care perspective that parallels and in ways intersects with trends in family medicine. Similar forces exist within each field: one more biomedical, the other more psychosocial. The psychosocially oriented sections of these two fields can provide the medical personnel for collaborative health care.

Such physicians accept the family (or household) as a basic unit of health care and also strongly consider other ecological health care factors—workplace, school, and community—whose relevance to people's health has been well-documented by now. They view health and illness systemically, following the continuum and hierarchy of natural and social systems (compare George Engel's writings), and can thus focus more on medicine's preventive and educative role, promoting health, not just treating disease. They can intervene at critical points in the life cycle of families, using therapy as well as medical skills.

Family-oriented medicine is growing because it meets the needs of Americans in a world that makes them feel alienated, frightened, and dismayed. In the midst of pain, isolation, and suffering, many people turn to their physicians. Physicians have always tried to promote comfort and security in times of stress, to deal with both the physical and the emotional aspects of people's distress. This can still be done, and even more effectively than is being done now.

Family Systems Medicine

Developments in systems theory in family medicine have brought us closer to what is now being called "family systems medicine" (compare the new eponymous journal). This is primary care but family-focused medicine that examines the diverse aspects of health and illness as they come up in the family. One of its main features is the collaboration between family medicine and the various family therapy fields. The growth of family systems medicine therefore can also abet moves towards collaborative health care.

Family Therapy

Family therapy, like family medicine but earlier, has grown enormously over the past decades. Now that it has attained maturity, the various family therapy groups have begun looking into questions of physical illness. Therapists and counselors see advantages in collaborating with physicians, especially as physicians can give them access to patients who need them.

Since its inception in the early 1950s, family therapy has developed models of family interaction which can help explain the diverse aspects of illness in a family context. Family therapists and counselors (I think here of the broadest linkages of family and marital therapists and counselors) are thus available to be the mental health personnel of collaborative health care (Bloch, 1982).

I am not concerned here with the different schools of family therapy, nor with the different degrees—both "terminal" and "non-terminal"—that therapists and counselors hold. Some conflicts between schools will be considered in Chapter 8. For now, let me say that family-oriented therapists and counselors not only exist in vast numbers, but they are showing more and more inclination to work alongside medical personnel in treating a variety of problems arising in medical settings—adjustment to illness, from both an individual and a family perspective; the treatment of illness in its family context; problems of chronic illness, problems of substance abuse in the family; helping a patient and his or her family deal with cancer; the question of noncompliance; the relationship of illness to life cycle stages, to stress, to family type. In addition, therapists and counselors work in a myriad of settings, from private offices to churches, from hospitals to community centers, from clinics to halfway houses, stress-reduction and biofeedback programs, and hospices.

Traditionally in the position of appealing to the more respected physicians for access to patients and families, therapists and counselors now have something to bargain with: they understand family dynamics better than physicians do; they are aware of communicative patterns better than physicians are; they can provide skills in a primary care physician's practice that no one else can provide, and that are helpful in managing on-going medical problems.

If family physicians practice collaboratively with family counselors and therapists, they can together care for the vast majority of people's everyday medical and psychological problems—and in an integrated fashion. There will be far less temptation to foster the "mind/body split."

Social Work

What I have said above about therapists and counselors holds, in great part, for many social workers today, practitioners whose main role is in providing counseling and therapy for patients and their families. Traditionally social workers have been attuned to the problems patients and families experience. They are familiar with the community and its resources. They are skilled at understanding problems of poverty, unemployment, housing, education, and of navigating the labyrinth of social bureaucracies. Some practices may well prefer linking up with a community-oriented social worker rather than with a mainly family therapy-oriented therapist. But more on this below.

Nursing

Nursing has a rich tradition of work with families in which an illness has occurred. Public health and community nursing have a long, respectable history. Visiting nurses are still the main health care professionals today who treat patients in their own homes. Nurses have traditionally been members of the family physician's office team. Many in recent years have taken a more independent position. Some have confronted the male-dominated medical hierarchy, and others have striven for a position in private practice on their own. Certainly, nursing has long been a repository of the psychosocial approach to health care. These professionals provide an important component to any collaborative health care team. Furthermore, nurses are often used to functioning as part of a team, and they are perceptive students of group/team process. Their discipline has amassed years of relevant primary care experience that they can bring to the collaborative health care effort.

Contributions from Other Fields

Social scientists have also entered this field. One thinks about the family stress project at the University of Minnesota, or of the efforts of the sociologist Tamara Hareven to deepen our historical understanding of the family as a social unit. The women's health and the alternative (holistic) health movements have also had an influence here. Wherever contributors from related social sciences have become involved with health care issues, they have made valuable contributions, and their continued presence as part of larger health care groups will be important in the coming years.

THE MODEL:
COLLABORATIVE FAMILY-ORIENTED HEALTH CARE

Collaborative family-oriented health care rests on collaboration between family physicians and family therapists or counselors. It treats patients' problems, both physical and emotional, in their social as well as biological context, and thus constitutes continuous comprehensive front-line health care.

The model is disarmingly simple. Family (or primary care) physicians and family therapists or counselors comprise the core personnel. These practitioners form teams or find other ways of combining their independence and togetherness. Allied health personnel can be added as needed. Such groups can be organized into fairly small, easily duplicable community-based practices. Between three and seven providers overall is enough, the internal growth of such groups occurring in a "cluster" fashion (see Figure 6.1). This could exist under a private practice model. It could be in government-funded clinics. It could be

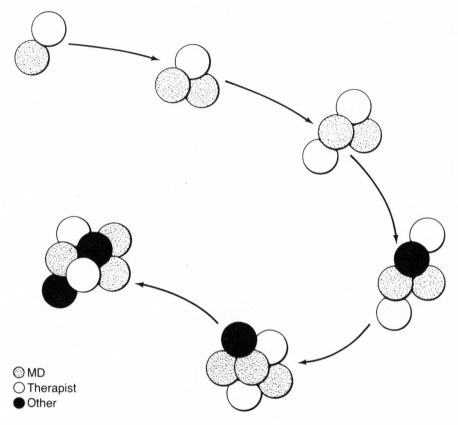

Figure 6.1 Growth of Staff in CHC Model.

organized in an HMO around small "modular" satellite clinics, each situated in a particular community, and each offering a local, personal form of primary medical care (see Figure 6.2).

Such collaborative practices might function as "gatekeepers" of care for HMOs or other programs. They would refer patients to specialists when necessary and would hospitalize patients in their affiliated community hospitals when that was necessary. If necessary, patients would have access to tertiary hospital care, too.

The model is applicable to almost any form of health care organization. The principle determinant is people's wanting to look at health care from a broader perspective. A team approach to health care can be utilized in teaching centers and training programs, where it has already been used; in community health centers (drawing back from a

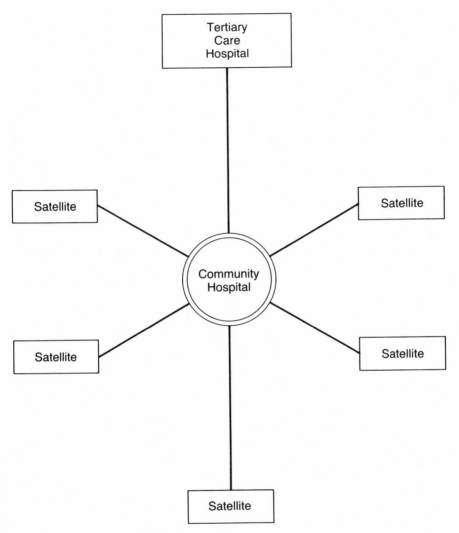

Figure 6.2   Satellite Clinics in CHC HMO.

tradition as old as the Peckham Experiment (Pearse and Crocker, 1943); in private practice, as Milt Seifert, Glen Aukerman, or the Northwest Family Medical Practice in Seattle have done it, and even in HMOs, which emphasize comprehensive and preventive care. Even under a socialized medical care system, such as England and Norway, primary care physicians and primary care counselors can work together.

In family medicine, as noted above, such collaboration is as old as the field itself. The first departments of family medicine brought together practicing family physicians who had left their practices to become teachers, and social science and therapy professionals who joined the new departments in order to train future family doctors in family matters, family dynamics, and a broader "systemic" perspective. Family medicine departments often harbor collaborative people whose academic teaching and private practice work both echo a collaborative inclination.

But one problem with collaborative teaching in family medicine residencies has been that, once residents leave the womb of the residency center, they often cannot practice what they've learned. This is because most family practice is still organized biomedically. Individual practitioners, perhaps with a physician assistant or a nurse, work in small offices. Two or three family physicians may form a group. The young family physicians who were trained by psychiatrists, therapists, and social workers usually have no one of that persuasion working with them when they enter practice. Economic incentives do not encourage it; it is hard to set up from scratch; and there are few models to learn from. Consequently, most of the new practitioners, even those who might want to work in collaboration with therapists, do not. Thus, visible working models of collaborative care are enormously important to the future of the field.

THE ARGUMENT RESTATED

Circumstances today differ from what prevailed in the 1960s. In 1965 there was no such thing as family medicine. And family therapy, still in its formative stages, had not yet begun to concern itself sharply with physical illness. Today, the factors have changed. Two large armies of primary health care providers stand ready to be joined. On the one hand is family medicine with tens of thousands of adherents. On the other hand is family therapy, increasingly concerned with physical illness and the family. Basic counseling can be joined with family practice into a model of health care that will keep family practice alive.

SETTINGS

Tertiary Care

For a long time, collaborative care has been available in large hospitals and clinics, as well as in university and training centers. The history of medical social work, liaison psychiatry, primary care nursing, and other such fields is intertwined with that of tertiary care hospitals and clinics. Typically, though, tertiary care treatment has been dominated by physicians, and much of the collaboration at that level has been between medical and psychiatric specialties. Disposition, however, and the wide variety of social service concerns, have often been left in the hands of the social service department; and these have included individual and family counseling over the past several decades.

Private Practice

In recent years collaborative work has been developing in the private sector (physicians' offices) as well as in HMOs. (More will be said regarding these in later chapters.) In a phrase, collaborative care in the private sector is relatively younger. It has been difficult for a variety of reasons (mainly the economic difficulties of obtaining reimbursement for the associated therapist), but there have been other problems as well:

• Reimbursement issues for the therapist/counselor: Payment comes from the insurance companies, Medicare, and Medicaid for their work.

• Time issues for the physician: The physician in private practice is reimbursed for direct service time, not for time spent sitting in with the counselor or for case-management discussions.

• Problems in conflicting outlook: Therapists and physicians have different training, different perspectives on the patient's problem, different mind-sets in general, and different priorities, based upon their actual daily routine. These create conflicts in professionally linked *style* and conflicts in *thinking*, that is, the way problems are framed (compare Bassoff, 1983 and Glenn et al., 1984). (For example, the physician who sees 750 patient visits a month may have a mind-set that does not incline him or her to initiate a discussion about one patient he has referred to the therapist. The therapist, who may be seeing 20 to 30 different people throughout the month, will be more inclined to initiate discussion about a patient with whom he is spending more time and whom he is getting to know more intimately than has the family physician. After all, it was for this that the referral was made in the first place.)

Forms of collaborative care in private practice are still in the early phases of their development. Nonetheless, they have already displayed an amazing variety.

Huygen's monograph (1978) describes collaborative work in the Netherlands. Johnston (1978) and Bhagat et al. (1979) describe such work in Great Britain. Comley (1973) describes work in Canada, as influenced by the McMaster model. The excellent volume by Miller (1983) discusses the advantages, as well as some drawbacks and difficulties of collaborative care.

Community Clinics

For many years, community clinics have been the most integrated, in terms of their staff. Nurses, physician assistants, social workers, therapists, and physicians of all types have all come together with social-minded administrators to help develop health programs especially concerned with a particular community. Collaborative care is no novelty to these people. Rather, their task todays is to keep their centers and clinics alive, and to preserve the community input and support they have amassed over time. Collaborative health care as a specific model can help situate some of these community clinics in the forefront of health care problems, a position many of them merit, but which few have been granted.

HMOs

Health maintenance organizations are the most vigorous and rapidly expanding forms of health care organization today. The main reason for their popularity and support is their insistence on providing care at a lower cost, while claiming to preserve high quality. Many of these programs achieve their savings by using different financial incentives—prepayment or capitation, as well as ways of sharing profits with the program's physician-managers. Some HMOs appear to emphasize a family perspective, and have a view of medical care as embracing the psychosocial dimensions described in previous chapters. Other HMOs sternly strip away or limit counseling services, claiming that this is one of the main ways they can contain their costs.

The HMOs that emphasize a holistic approach, and that practice preventive medicine as a way of holding costs down in the long run, will be most open, in the coming years, to the idea of collaborative health care. They will find it less expensive to cover counseling than to ignore it, and they will find it less expensive to have in-house, collaborative counselors than to subcontract therapy services with outside providers or clinics. Such programs offer tremendous potential for gathering scientific data on the effects of therapy intervention and counseling services on the overall health cost dollar, as well as on the public health. If HMOs can lock in their panels of patients, treat them, and keep records about what happens to their members' health status, they will affect national health care policy. This challenge for the HMOs involves their taking the long- not the short-term view, and following a broad bio-psychosocial rather than a limited biomedical perspective on health and illness and on the services they will offer to promote the one and cope with the other.

PART
TWO

SEVEN

Collaborative Health Care in Practice

All areas of life affect people's health. It follows therefore that understanding health goes beyond the simple question of deciding whether one is ill or not. Physicians who would transcend the biomedical model must learn to look into the variegated aspects of people's experience. They must share this task with others, too, and learn to work with counselors or therapists whose skills complement their own. People often consult physicians with a physical symptom, hoping mainly to find a kind and sympathetic heart, get some understanding and advice, and encounter someone with whom they can talk things over. More people initially visit their family physician for emotional problems than go to psychiatrists or counselors. Will primary care physicians be capable of dealing with these people in distress? Collaborative practice is a natural way for them to meet the needs of such patients, who bring a wide range of problems to their physician.

Collaborative health care efforts have thus far taken a number of different forms. This chapter describes some of them.

In private practice, guidelines have generally been molded by physician dominance. The medical practice usually antedates collaborative efforts, and the physician is the hub of medical care. Sensing that additional skills and personnel might be useful for dealing with his or her patients' needs, the physician then employs a therapist, social worker, or counselor. The latter is seen as ancillary to the practice as a whole, and is expected to thank the physician for giving him or her access to a wide variety of patients. Most of the problems of collaboration in primary health care, in fact, flow from this structure, in which physicians, naturally assuming the leadership role, view the counselor as simply another specialist to whom they are referring their patient for adjunctive treatment, while they keep control of the situation as a whole in their own hands.

Physicians interested in building a collaborative practice must therefore learn to cooperate better. Often, this means spending more time with their counselor colleagues. They will have to define responsibilities more clearly. In addition, in setting up their practices, they will have to cope with the limitations of their actual situation. They will have to accept the restraints and resources of their community. For example, it may be difficult for them to find the ideal family-oriented Ph.D. therapist, so they might have to hire a social worker with a keen interest in family counseling instead. A physician may want to hire a female counselor, but may have to settle for a male instead, because this particular male therapist more suitably shares the physician's basic orientation. It is always hard to find an ideal "other."

The question of fit between colleagues is critical to working well together. Some factors that affect this are: (1) congruence of personal styles, (2) shared political beliefs and social/moral values, (3) agreement on the importance of psychosocial factors in people's illness experience, (4) shared attitudes towards the importance of listening to people's problems in living, (5) attitudes towards cooperation, (6) and shared degree of openness to criticism. These factors notwithstanding, the most basic ingredient in working well together is clear communication about who is responsible for what, and how.

CURRENT FORMS OF ORGANIZATION OF COLLABORATIVE HEALTH CARE

Private Practice

Private practice is still the predominent mode of practice in the United States today. Collaborative care in a private practice setting has taken a wide variety of forms, running a gamut from the physician as the center and the organizer of the practice to the physician and counselor as partners in a somewhat equal endeavor.

Traditional model:
The physician refers to a therapist who is not in the same practice

Nellie Grose, a Houston family physician, works collaboratively with therapists by referral. She asserts that all therapists are not the same, and argues that all family therapists are not the same either. She holds certain criteria for therapists with whom she works. Foremost among these is that the therapist must have a systemic and strategic sense.

> I began to learn about different models and different therapists, and got to know most importantly their orientation. The way I select them in referral truly depends upon the needs of the patient. To be more specific, there are patients who might want a young therapist. Gender might be important. Religious background may be important. These are some of the factors I take into consideration. First of all I have to understand their theoretical orientation. Secondly, communication is extremely important: there is feedback in both directions. And, thirdly, the interests of the patient comes first.
>
> I think I work best with people with a strategic approach. First it lends itself better to improving the doctor-patient relationship, which is the most important part of the encounter. Secondly, it regards the patient as the most important person. And thirdly it provides me the opportunity to take charge and take responsibility for change.

Grose's way of making a referral shows how she sticks closely to her colleague. Even though the therapist may be across town, Grose manages to focus on the collaborative issues she feels most strongly about:

> When I make a referral I do call the therapist and speak to the therapist in person about the question I want answered or the problem I'm having with the nature of the consultation and some of the questions the patient might have about the therapist, let's say "herself" this time. After the therapist then has the phone number and the name and in the event the patient does not call up within a week, it is not unusual for the therapist to call the patient. We often find it increases the compliance because if a therapist is strategic in her approach, this would often get the patient in for consultation. It is very customary for the therapist, after the first consultation, to give me some feedback on the phone. I like a phone report because it provides me with a lot of information and I can often learn from the feedback, and that is one good way of learning more about any kind of referral, be it pediatrics, medicine, gynecology. In subsequent visits—it may be right away, it may be after two visits—progress is always given back to me. One of the things I always ask is what must I not do to sabotage the referral process, because often family members can call you in a crisis and that crisis may be the very thing that is necessary to create change, so I often find it important to know the things I must not do.

This form of practice actually has many advantages. First, physicians with limited office space may select it, because they don't have to build a new office or relocate. Finding a therapist elsewhere in town also permits physicians to choose the most suitable therapists for their colleagues: they don't have to choose from among the smaller pool of therapists willing to move into a physician's space. In addition, they can maintain an interprofessional, not an employer-employee relationship. For the therapist, such an arrangement protects the security of having his or her own practice. The therapist does not have to move into the physician's office, does not have to be paid by the physician, and is not dependent on a single physician for his or her clients.

Collaborative, but traditional:
Physicians have therapist colleagues in their practice,
but are clearly the leaders of the working group

In many primary care practices, physicians have hired a full- or part-time counselor to meet their patients' psychosocial needs. Pediatricians may hire a nurse educator—the U.S. equivalent of the British *health visitor*—and internists or family physicians may hire a counselor. The core of this model is that physicians are still the main providers of care. After all, they argue, their practice is basically medical; the great majority of patients come because of some kind of physical malaise or physical symptom and remain in the practice through their developing relationship to the physician. The counselor is seen as ancillary, someone the physician has brought in to help in the overall task, and to whom the physician sends clients, often even indicating just what form of counselling they should receive.

In Milton Seifert's Excelsior, Minnesota practice, for example, the "therapist" is a health coordinator, a counselor in problems of living who has been trained in the Alcoholics Anonymous "Twelve Step" program, which Seifert has adopted to fit the needs of patients going through all kinds of stress:

> [I took] the AA twelve step program and appl[ied] it to the lives of people, to the acceptance of cancer, diabetes, heart disease, because that seemed to be the same dynamics as acceptance of alcoholism. The management of stress so that you don't have to drink is the management of stress whether it has anything to do with alcohol or not. . . . My idea was to [have the counselor] teach people something basic, which I could hook back into as the physician (Seifert, Interview, 1985).

Seifert maintains control of his medical practice. When he wishes to refer a patient to his counselor, he writes out a prescription telling the counselor what particular basic approaches he wants him to go over with the patient. Part of this has to do with Seifert's notion of diagnosis. Rather than diagnose "mental illnesses," Seifert tends to regard many problems in living as problems of faulty, inadequate skills. The counselor is really an educator, a teacher. In order to get patients to identify the skills they need to learn, Seifert relies on what he terms the "language of negotiation." Through this process, he works with the patient to reach a mutually acceptable, nonpejorative description of the problem. Once he reaches a mutual diagnosis with his patients, he can then refer them to the counselor for specific guidance. It is important to understand how he does not refer patients to his health coordinator for treatment of mental illnesses or psychiatric problems; and he does not look upon the counselor's work as "therapy": "One of the important parts is that we wanted this to be educative and not counselling. We drew the line at advising people. We just wanted to teach them some skills, support them in solving their problems, keep them going, and try to stay away from things like insight or even various kinds of psychological beliefs."

The language of negotiation includes such terms as "independence/dependence imbalance," "patient-role difficulty," "impulse control deficiency," and "sensitive person." The terms are nonpejorative and can be discussed with the patient in order to reach a contract for counseling by consensus. Seifert's notion of therapy, at least insofar as it exists in a family practice, is thus thoroughly didactic. Seifert does not see problems as "psychological," but rather as problems of deficient skill, inadequate education, and so on. This permits him to offer what might be called "reframed" diagnoses to patients, who can begin to accept their own shortcomings and enter treatment for them, because the labels make sense to them. Seifert has in fact shown that his terms are both easier to understand and less pejorative than standard psychiatric terms (speech at STFM March meeting, 1985):

> We set out with the intention of creating a language both providers and patients could understand. We collaborated with our patients in the process. For example, we looked at the person who's too dependent, or too independent, or like the alcoholic, who's independent where he should be dependent and vice versa; or the person who can't walk but isn't willing to do the things he or she can do, like learn[ing] to transfer and take care of themselves. These are people who are willing to do what they cannot and unwilling to do what they can, and it's very helpful to have a conceptual handle on them. 'Independence/dependence imbalance' is the term we ended up with. . . .

Another example might be the non-compliant patient who can be called a lot of names, but the term we use is 'patient-role difficulty.' I say to him, 'Do you have difficulty being the patient? Is it hard for you to go to a doctor? That could be for any one of a variety of reasons, and you have a right to be that way, but it is a problem, and we need to put it on the problem list.'

Once the patient has begun seeing the health coordinator, Seifert continues to keep tabs on the process. When the basics have been taught, he will bring the patient and family members back in for an evaluation. The health coordinator has input to this process, too. In doing this, Seifert has found that almost all the patients he refers to the counselor wind up keeping the appointment. Furthermore, he likes the counselor's being directly responsible to himself. It gives him the sense of an integrated practice, which he commands.

Practices such as Seifert's provide the advantages of integrating on-site counselling—as well as other useful adjunctive health modalities—into a general medical practice. The physician's central position is not threatened, and the physician's aura can be used to promote patients' accepting the new personnel. The physician can also bring in a wide variety of health professionals and direct them to follow his or her own protocols for treatment, thus ensuring an overall integrated approach to the practice. On the other hand, counselors and other health professionals can gain the benefits of having a ready-made clientele and (usually) the security of a salaried position. They do relinquish their autonomy, however, as well as some sense of professional control. Professional boundaries in such a practice must be carefully negotiated.

Collaborative: Physicians not only work with a therapist in their practice, they also learn counseling skills themselves

A currently popular form of collaborative care has a physician and a counselor/therapist working within the same practice and both providing counseling services. Often, the physician still retains leadership, but at times the two will work conjointly with regard to making decisions. Usually the physician is the original practitioner—that is, it was his or her practice first—but has over the course of time become convinced that s/he needs a counselor to provide the kind of extended care the practice needs, attention to the psychosocial dimensions of patients' illness. The physician then searches for an appropriate therapist to bring into the practice. This occurs as a pediatrician hires a nurse practitioner with particular skills in helping teach young mothers about issues in the care of young children. It occurs as a busy family practitioner in a working-class town hires a social worker to help with his patients' many social and economic problems. It occurs as a family physician becomes attuned to the high incidence of psychosocial problems in his or her practice and wishes to bring a counselor or family therapist aboard to help these patients and their families work their problems out.

Doherty and Baird. An excellent introduction to this kind of collaborative work is presented by William Doherty and Macaran Baird's *Family Therapy and Family Medicine* (1983). The senior author is a clinical psychologist with training in family systems theory, the junior a family physician. Having worked together in practice for some time, they then both became faculty members at the University of Oklahoma School of Medicine.

The book presents a theoretical model for the collaborative work between these two disciplines, then devotes several chapters to illustrating work with particular problems: noncompliance, substance abuse, depression, anxiety, and sexual difficulties. It begins with the case for a family orientation in health care. The authors then present a model for the "primary care of families." This systemic approach, emphasizing that "the physician is part of system" (p. 12), involves (1) understanding the "therapeutic triangle in family practice"—the relationship between the patient, the physician, and the family (medical practice is not "dyadic"); (2) assessing the stages in the primary care of families—observation, assessment, contracting, referring or treating—and (3) examining the options for the treatment of the common psychosocial problems encountered in family (primary care) practice. To depict the latter, Doherty and Baird provide an amazing graph one axis of which expresses the level of the treatment unit—individual, couple, family, community—while the other describes the type of counseling received—ad hoc primary care counseling, repeated primary care counseling, specialized therapy.

The book is buttressed with a discussion of rudimentary family systems theory, especially the work of Salvador Minuchin, however its strength lies not in the theory it presents but in its feel for clinical practice. Following their theoretical discussion, the authors discuss actually observing and assessing families in practice. Their discussion includes a list of "red flags" suggesting family dysfunction—clinical pearls that any family physician will understand. The subsequent chapter continues examining "real work" by studying how to form a therapeutic contract that involves the whole family (not just one family member or the identified patient). This latter discussion considers the difficulties of translating the somatic symptom into a biopsychosocial understanding—for the patient, as well as the physician. Later chapters deal with the critical issues of referring or treating and the basics of counseling families.

Doherty and Baird's model promotes two concepts: first, that the family physician can be trained to counsel families through many of the common psychosocial problems people experience, and second, that a family therapist can function as a specialist adjunct to family practice (for those patients/families whose problems are beyond the family physician's skill).

Regarding the first of these points, Doherty, in a later article (1985, p. 132) comments:

> A main hindrance to family interventions in health care has been the notion that only trained family therapists are equipped to help families experiencing difficulties. In the Doherty and Baird model, however, family interventions can be viewed on a continuum from primary care to specialized therapy, with most health professionals functioning toward the primary care end of the continuum. . . . Basically, the more severe and chronic psychosocial problems are best handled by trained therapists, whereas many health-related and life cycle issues could be handled by a primary care health professional who has appropriate training.

Counseling in primary care has four main functions: education, prevention, support, and challenge. Education teaches families about health issues such as coping with illness, diet, and child rearing. Prevention helps prevent illness through anticipatory guidance. Support refers to helping families cope with the demands of health problems and other stressors. Challenge involves an effort to help restructure dysfunctional families through simple measures or a therapy referral. Primary care counseling is carefully distinguished from family therapy, which is "aimed at major family system overhaul or at least a decisive breakthrough in serious family dysfunction" (p. 89). The authors' concern for the training and practice of family physicians can be shown in their focus on training—for physicians. The family physician can learn "different levels" of skill in working with families. Some family physicians become so interested in doing family therapy that they take up higher training in it and become skilled at doing it. Others learn to work with a compatible therapy collaborator.

In his later article, Doherty further develops this notion of "levels of expertise"—a concept very appropriate for helping family physicians understand what they can and cannot do, and where the boundaries of their field lie. His notion of levels of expertise echoes the McMaster model which has also been used to train family physicians to intervene successfully in the life events of their patients. Doherty organizes the "levels of physician involvement with families" by several parameters—the knowledge base required for such work, the need for personal development (read "awareness"), the skills to be learned. Level 1 is "minimal emphasis on family." At this level the physician deals with families "only as necessary" (p. 134). Emphasis is on the individual patient. Level 2 involves "ongoing medical information and advice." It requires an understanding of the family-patient-physician triangle, and it brings the physician to see the individual patient in a family context. Family members are used both as sources of information and as recipients of care and information. Level 3 is called "feelings and support." If the shift from Level 1 to Level 2 represents "a new awareness that families are important parts of biomedical health care," (p. 133), then the further shift to Level 3 represents "a shift from a primarily biomedical paradigm to a more humanistic one that emphasizes affective care of patients and their families in addition to treating and preventing medical illness" (p. 133). Finally, the shift to Level 4, "systematic assessment and planned intervention," represents a shift to a systemic way of looking at things. It is at this level that family therapy per se takes place. Doherty then goes on to comment on what levels of expertise and involvement might be required in family medicine training.

I feel the continuum is absolutely true, but I sense that the distinction between primary care counseling and family therapy evades the central issue of professional turf. All families have difficulties. All physicians counsel. The line between counseling and therapy is imprecise. Sometimes one counsels and the family changes. Sometimes therapy's goal is making small changes. Is the difference that a therapist uses therapy techniques? (Suppose a physician unwittingly used therapy techniques while counseling?) Is the difference in the skills learned, and in the capacity to conceptualize the problem? (Suppose some physician moves instinctively to correct and cure a problem, even though s/he cannot conceptualize what s/he did.) The confusion is magnified by therapy converts in family medicine who become true hybrids and who actually do want to practice family therapy several hours a week. I think the line between the two activities is in fact blurry. For those at either end of the spectrum, to be sure, there is much less blur. But for those toward the middle, I think there's a good deal of blur. Similarly, Doherty's attempt to differentiate Levels 2, 3, and 4 seems a bit forced.

I think Doherty and Baird's main aim is to reassure people and safeguard turf. They reassure therapists that physicians won't try to "do therapy," while letting physicians feel free to go ahead and "counsel." In a way, this is playing with words. The authors want to push family medicine toward a more systemic, less strictly biomedical model, and this cannot but involve some anxiety on the part of both traditional physicians and traditional therapists. Doherty and Baird aim at giving family physicians permission to deal with family problems; they also aim at bringing family systems thinking more closely into the acceptable mainstream of family medicine, especially at a time when family medicine is tilting back toward traditional general practice. Problems with their model, certainly less worrisome than the problems preexisting it—that is, with the biomedical model—involve some physicians' misunderstanding the complexity of family therapy and presuming arrogantly that they have become experts overnight. But this is a failing of physicians in general, trainees especially, and most enthusiasts. The effects of time and a few hard failures work wonders to correct unrealistic assumptions.

Christie-Seely. The family physician may learn to do therapy and/or work with therapists, but the main focus is "working with families in primary care." Janet Christie-Seely (1984), a Canadian family practitioner and teacher, takes a similar course to Doherty and Baird's (1983). Her commitment to a systems approach is evident in her first chapters. These define the family system, discuss the "healthy" family, and point out the importance of the family life cycle to its members' health. Ensuing chapters look at other systems in which family life occurs—the community, culture, and values.

Her attempt to distinguish "working with the family" from "family therapy" seems more successful than Doherty's:

> The phrase "working with the family," originally coined by Dr. Yves Talbot, denotes working in a collaborative relationship with families over time with a focus on promotion of health and treatment of illness. This contrasts with family therapy, in which there is a contract for change in the family system (p. xvii).

Such a distinction seems appropriate to primary care and makes it clearer why primary care professionals need to know the family as a system, without turning them all into family counselors or therapists. Here, Christie-Seely leaves all claim to therapy, counselling, and so on, to the therapists, and (modestly!) contents herself with the task of merely "working with" the family. Such an ingenuous disclaimer serves as prelude to a carefully wrought presentation of what such modest "work" can accomplish. It is important that Christie-Seely avoids disputing turf and focuses instead on promoting health and treating illness—terms both broad and narrow enough to accommodate much diversity. (And, if, in the course of promoting health, one helps a family to change, so much the better, she seems to be saying.)

All in all, however, Christie-Seely does not deal much with collaborative care. Her focus is almost all on the primary care physician or nurse. "Rarely," she states, "[will] a family . . . need or request more intensive intervention" (p. 252), by which she means family therapy. When there is such a need, she is content with advising a referral to a known and qualified family therapist, although she expresses interest (p. 256) in practices in which a family therapist has joined a group of physicians. She backs away from advocating a team approach or even the closer collaboration Doherty and Baird encourage.

Physicians and therapists in the same practice, defining their degree of collaboration as they go. Family physician works with therapist in office, mainly by referral. This working arrangement exists at many different locations. It is the type of arrangement at our own Everett Family Practice and it has been pursued by the Northwest Family Medicine group in Seattle. It has sprung up in private practice in Georgia, Texas, Virginia, and probably in every other state in the United States. The basis for such work is a collaboration between health care professionals, based on the particular features of the practice—rural/urban, affluent/working class, large/small, group/solo—as well as on the specific disciplines represented, the professionals' overall orientation, and their personalities, as well as the unique process that takes place in each different practice.

In our practice, for example, our therapists are Linda Atkins, who has an M.A. and training in family therapy, and Martin Cohen, who has both a Ph.D. in clinical psychology and further training in family therapy. Both have a keen appreciation of family systems. These therapists bill for their own services, but they pay rent for the use of space.

Most of their referrals come from the family practice, but some come from without. Collaborative meetings occur each week, but therapists and physicians usually work in parallel, not in the same place at the same time.

Other practices involve the physician's (or physician's corporation's) taking a percentage of the therapist's fee for the privilege of working together. The therapist is in essence paying tribute for the access to patients the physician(s) guarantee. Or, perhaps, the therapist might be on a salary, with either the physician or the practice billing for his or her services. There are many variations on this theme.

The question of who's in charge is fascinating to tease out. In our practice we sometimes opt for giving the therapist a great deal of control over the entire health care treatment of patients they are treating. In some cases, this means the therapist is playing a decisive role in dealing with the *medical* management of their patients. At other times we insist on very close collaboration, so that the patient (and/or family) will not "split" the physician and the counselor. We do this when patients are experiencing physical symptoms as an expression of their therapy treatment, and we also do it when patients appear chronically obsessed with their physical illnesses and unable to cope with their other day-to-day feelings (depressed hypochondriacs, for example).

We have found that the physician can be a tremendous resource to the therapist's treatment efforts, especially if the therapist tells the physician how to behave around certain critical issues. Robert Singer, for example, asks our therapists to:

> Tell me what to do. You're working with the patient and the family, much more intensively than I am. I may see seven hundred patient visits in a month, while you may see thirty different people in the same time span. So tell me what you want me to do. Balint says the physician is a 'drug.' Look at me that way yourself—as a drug, a 'tool.' I'm a therapeutic resource. Instruct me, use me the way you think I'd be most effective. Do you want me to encourage a particular person to be independent? Do you want me to help a daughter get closer to her father, and less dependent on her mother? Tell me.

In the Northwest Family Medicine practice in Seattle, Larry Mauksch, a counselor, works with two family physicians, William Phillips and Scott Stevens. They describe their relationship (Mauksch and Phillips, 1985) as "integrating professional practices . . . a complex, collegial relationship." Phillips feels that the presence of a counselor in the office "says something about our commitment to see health care as going beyond the medical model. . . . This encourages the patient, as well as ourselves, to take a broader view of the therapeutic modalities that might be helpful."

Discussions about mutual patients are carried out informally so that care is coordinated. The counselor bills for his own services, but he pays rent to the practice. This arrangement has been so successful that Mauksch and Phillips have twice given a workshop on "Integrating Professional Practices" to people who wanted to learn about their model and their experiences.

In this variant of the collaborative model, the therapist(s) and physician(s) can spend as much time together as they want. They can meet regularly, as we do in Everett, or they can catch one another informally when the need arises. Communication takes place in the patient's (family's) chart, too, if both counselor and physician use the same chart. In Seattle, the sheets in the charts are color-coded by provider. If they want, the therapist and physician can see patients or families together; they can observe one another, hold conjoint meetings with a family, or divide the work to be done between themselves as they see fit.

The basic requirements for such an arrangement to succeed are having open communication and setting aside time to get together. If the physician is too busy to see the counselor, a hierarchy develops in which the therapist has to petition the physician for time. Such a relationship can engender hidden resentments.

In a collaborative practice, the professionals must be able to explore their own expectations, need, and readiness for work. A physician who works 55 hours a week may not be overly sympathetic to a therapist who chooses to work 30 hours a week but who wants to make as much income in 30 hours as the physician does in 55. The physician makes more money per hour, but has to spend 50 percent of it for office overhead; the therapist makes less but has much less overhead. In the same vein, a hard-working therapist may resent the physician's capacity to make twice as much money. These very basic considerations must be placed "on the table," open for discussion. What Phillips calls the "fit" of the counselor and physician becomes important, too. Nothing goes further to cement a relationship across interdisciplinary lines than shared values, shared perspective, and compatible personalities.

The family physician and therapist work collaboratively, actually seeing patients together

Barry Dym, a skilled family therapist, and one of the founders of the Cambridge Family Institute, has evolved a collaborative model quite different from what others have proposed. Rejecting the notion that a therapist working with a physician must be in a consultative position, Dym advocates the new role of a "primary care therapist," an actual working partner of the primary care physician. Dym envisages the family physician and the primary care therapist forming a team, and both meeting patients and their families at intake (and other occasions). The team assesses the problem collaboratively, decides upon a treatment plan, and then divides up the work.

Dym has put this idea into practice in a provisional way by spending Thursday afternoons in the office of a family physician, Ron Backer of Winchester, Massachusetts. Working along at Backer's pace—about four or five patients an hour—Dym sits in the room as the physician goes through his history and physical exam, and then intervenes as the psychosocial, dynamic issues become clear:

> I begin by observing: everything, really. I listen to the patient. I watch what's going on in the patient's relationship with Ron. Mainly I look for the psychological and interpersonal context of the presenting problem. . . . Within about three minutes I can start to see an interactional pattern. I will then tend to make the move that links the presenting problem to the interactional context. All this happens in an informal way, while Ron is conducting his examination.

In Dym's opinion, such work calls for a new kind of therapist. Instead of focusing on the special work of psychotherapy, the primary care therapist is more concerned with observing and assessing, with perceiving the patterns going on in a family and intervening to clarify or challenge them.

> The reason I feel the need to experiment now, before separating, is that functional divisions between doctors and therapists are premature. When doctors refer psychosomatic patients to the therapist, it can simply rigidify the mind/body split. The same can be true for referrals to the therapist for neurotic or behavioral problems. These arrangements don't challenge the basic assumptions which permeate the field. We need time to look at every case, from an integrative angle, which requires two people with an equal stand and equal experience, not someone who's in charge and someone who's not, in order even to *begin* to say whose skills are most relevant, for what and when.

Dym feels that this new primary care therapist needs different skills from the psychotherapist-specialist. Since most of his or her work is going to be in the realm of observation and assessment, quick intervention, and brief treatment, the primary care therapist will need a blend of talents:

A primary care therapist should be trained in brief, strategically-oriented, problem-solving psychotherapy. There are other skills which have nothing to do with family therapy *per se* which are also essential. You have to know something about relaxation, meditation, biofeedback, and perhaps hypnosis. You have to know something about using guided imagery, as is done with cancer patients. You've got to develop a systematic approach to prevalent medical dilemmas like compliance. And, in the same way as family physicians will want to know more about psychotherapy, therapists who work in this area will want to know more about the physiological aspects of illness. It's truly not a family therapist we're talking about, but a systemically-oriented therapist who can see the biological, psychological and social world, and the community as a whole.

Such a model is challenging and audacious. It undercuts the usual pattern of medical dominance and medical hierarchy by insisting that the therapist (or systems thinker) has equally critical skills to bring to the health care encounter. These skills have taken years of training and experience to acquire, and they complement the skills the physician has learned through his or her own training. Dym throws down a gauntlet to those who advocate a collaborative model: He asserts that the collaborative team should be together at the crucial starting point, the point of diagnosing and defining the problem, more so than later on down the line when therapy is simply a matter of triage. The latter approach rests on the physician's defining the problem. Dym's model calls on the physician and the therapist to collaborate in investigating the problem, looking at the data, and defining the scope of treatment. He feels the primary care team does its best work in defining the problem before it becomes rigidified and hardened in the biomedical model, a notion that echoes Michael Balint's view of "negotiating" the diagnosis with the patient.

Dym's model, described in greater detail in a later article (Dym and Berman, 1986) breaks with the prevailing medical notions, reaching beyond them to a broader systemic perspective. Features that his model provide, which are not present in some of the other, looser forms of collaborative care include:

• In usual collaboration, the mind/body split is subtly maintained, because the counselor or therapist is a specialist, a professional whose "turf" is the area of emotional and family problems, while the referring physician remains concerned with overall medical triage, the overall picture, and biomedical procedures. In Dym's model, both professionals develop a data base, perspective, and plan together, utilizing one another's skills to come up with a truly conjoint plan. This means that mind and body problems are integrated, not split off.

• In usual collaboration, the physician is the dominant professional. The therapist or counselor follows the physician's lead. In Dym's model, the therapist and the physician are professionals of equal stature working together.

• In usual collaboration, the skills of the counselor or therapist are applied to the psychosocial problem at hand. In Dym's model, the therapist's skills are used to focus on the most common of medical problems, the behavior and communications that emerge during the routine office visit.

• Dym's model pursues the "strategic" outlook common to a particular school of contemporary family therapy (compare Lynn Hoffman, 1981).

Dym says that every medical patient he sees has psychosocial issues that he, as a trained family therapist, feels he can address in a helpful way. Not only is the development and occurrence of illness linked to psychosocial factors, not only is the patient's presenting behavior linked to psychosocial factors, but the entire question of *managing* the patient's problem, whether it involves life-style counseling (smoking, obesity), matters of compliance, or the impact of the illness of the patient upon the patient's family is something the therapist or counselors has special expertise in addressing. Furthermore, the family therapist may be able to help the physician perceive the family's patterns of illness, much as Peachey and Huygen have described, so that the collaborative team can focus in on them and their significance.

Initially, Dym began working with Ron Backer, in the latter's family practice. For a time, the two of them explored the model of working together. Now he and his colleagues are beginning to train others. He has recently announced a series of courses to be given at the Cambridge Family Institute for therapists who wish to work with physicians, and for physicians who wish to understand more about the techniques and purpose of family therapy.

Dym's ideas and practice are evolving, and what might be said in 1986 as I write these words may no longer be so in 1987 or later when these words are being read. One set of comments must be raised, however, which all focus around the basic question: How can it work financially?

How, one must ask, is the therapist reimbursed for the time spent with the family and the physician? In a private practice model, this raises the problem of co-billing. Insurance companies, as is well known these days, are more and more concerned with cutting their costs. To do this, they are often refusing to pay more than one provider for simultaneous services, and they also refuse to pay for services they do not consider medically necessary. It has become increasingly difficult for physicians and therapists to obtain payment for services rendered for medical diagnosis; it will be even more difficult to get money from the insurance companies for nonurgent, elective, or screening psychotherapy (even worse, *family* therapy purposes).

Many Medicaid programs that cover care for the indigent will not pay a counselor or therapist for psychotherapy services unless he or she is either a psychiatrist or connected with an approved mental health clinic or center. This means that any therapist in a private practice setting who sees Medicaid patients will not be reimbursed for his or her services. Thus, simultaneous therapist/medical practice in a private practice setting will involve some juggling of funds. The physician may actually have to split his or her fee with the therapist, or vice versa. Or the two of them may have to agree to lower their own life-styles and incomes in order to practice in this most collaborative way. If the therapists received most of their salary by doing psychotherapy, of course, they would be able to free up some time for sitting-in with the physician. But this is precisely what Barry Dym wants to avoid in creating a separate kind of "primary-care therapist." He doesn't want the therapists spending all their time doing therapy, but rather working side by side with the family physician. One other option, of course, is for the insurance companies to begin to understand the value of preventive health visits, and to reimburse for such treatment. But this would mean a complete restructuring of the fee scale in private practice, just at a time when services are being even more tightly controlled.

Dym recognizes this problem. Recently (1986), he has commented:

> Then there is the question of how I get paid. This is no problem when people are covered by insurance, since I am a licensed psychologist. I can bill for 25 minute sessions. But I cannot bill for Medicare and Medicaid, and I cannot bill for some of the pre-paid health plans, such as Bay State, which are highly prejudicial towards all but physicians. I am per-

fectly willing to absorb this loss during this experimental period, but for others depending on this collaboration as their main income source, careful selection of patients for whom collaboration is possible will be a must—at least until third party payers are more enlightened. It is clear that all of us interested in close collaborative models will have to make the case, probably through research, that it is cost-effective.

The problem becomes much less acute when one leaves the private practice setting. In an HMO, for example, all health care providers are paid on salary, or by some combination of salary-with-incentive. Their work time is capable of being structured to meet the needs of the patients, as the HMO defines them. Thus, if the HMO feels that primary care teams would actually decrease its overall health care cost outlay—through early identification of at-risk situations and burgeoning problems, and early intervention, which might diminish the later cost of more serious illness and emotional disturbance—it might very well set such teams in operation. It is no accident, therefore, that Dym has been approached by at least one large HMO to inquire into the feasibility of his ideas in their program. Certainly, more studies need to be done to see if the above assumptions are correct, but this can be done if an HMO wishes to investigate.

Such an approach would look at health maintenance from a family and social perspective. It would focus on recognition of maladaptive family patterns, "signs of trouble," and the emotional factors that accompany all diseases and that condition the patient's response to the physician's treatment. It is an approach that moves strikingly away from the usual episodic, crisis-oriented model of care that prevails today.

Among all the collaborative models, Dym's most challenges prevailing views, even those among procollaborative practice people. For this reason, one would like to see some HMO, some university group, some foundation give this model a chance to prove its ultimate cost-effectiveness and health-promotional capacity by funding a long-term (10 or 15 year) study of its effectiveness.

Holistic health collaboration

Yet another form of private practice collaboration follows the outline of the holistic health movement. A good example of this form is William Manahan's Mankato, Minnesota practice, especially its newly formed Wellness Center.

Manahan shares the perspectives of the holistic health movement—its focus on health rather than illness, its multidisciplinary orientation, and its concern with diet, exercise, nutrition, and stress management. The following excerpts are from a booklet describing the Wellness Center:

> The Wellness Center . . . exists to assist individuals in attaining optimum comprehensive health.
>
> For some, this may mean a program aimed at renewal. For persons suffering hypertension, heart disease, excessive stress or "burnout," or those in transition due to a death, divorce or other loss, changes in behavior, living habits and attitudes may be sought. . . .
>
> In each individuals case, the aim of the Center's comprehensive program is not only to help resolve immediate problems, but also to help establish healthier life-style patterns (Spring Calendar, 1985, p. 3).

The staff of the Wellness Center includes a director with a doctorate in Sacred Theology, several mental health therapists, a biofeedback therapist, a dietician, a personal health planner (B.S. in nursing, further training in psychiatric/mental health nursing), a relaxation/stress management nurse, and a physical fitness coordinator.

This staff not only treats patients. They also give lecture sessions, day-long workshops, and one- to five-day resident programs (retreats) on topics related to the management of stress in everyday life. They provide evening talks—"Sodium Smarts," "Protecting your Heart," "Delightful Dining," "Family Satisfaction," and so on—and other talks on a wide variety of nutritional, family-focused, and stress-management topics. In this, they are one of the several holistic health centers that have sprung up across the country, mainly in the suburbs and among the middle classes, but also in other areas as well. (For more about this orientation, compare *Mind, Body, and Health: Towards an Integral Medicine*, edited by James S. Gordon, Dennis T. Jaffe, and David E. Bresler [New York: Human Sciencies Press, 1984] ; John H. Milsum, *Health, Stress, and Illness: A Systems Approach* [New York: Praeger, 1984] ; and Kenneth R. Pelletier, *Holistic Medicine* [New York: Delacorte, 1979]. For a critique of this movement, compare Larry Sirott and Howard Waitzkin's article "Holism and self-care: Can the individual succeed where society fails?" in Victor W. Sidel and Ruth Sidel [eds.] *Reforming Medicine: Lessons of the Last Quarter Century* [New York: Pantheon, 1984].)

Under this (holistic) model, medical care is redefined as wellness care, and the emphasis is on learning better life-style, practicing preventive medicine, and learning ways of reducing stress. The physician employs a wide number of ancillary health professionals, especially those utilizing physical (somatic) techniques.

Such an approach enables the physician to bring many collegial health professionals into the family practice setting. It also makes it easier to educate patients about the effects of stress on their health and to help them develop healthier habits. Counselors, nutritionists, and physical therapists can contribute their own special skills to the whole treatment of the individual and the family, without necessitating that the physician become a "jack-of-all-trades" him- or herself. The main problem with this kind of care appears to be paying for it. That is, its cost is often not reimbursable by the insurance companies; its practitioners often cannot accept Medicaid; the elderly are not a major portion of this kind of care; and its appeal tends to be limited to the more affluent sections of the population. Interestingly, perhaps owing to the antimedical bias of many of the holistic health movement's advocates, in our rubric of collaborative models, this model is one that often tends *not* to be physician-centered.

Public Settings

Collaborative care has been practiced in public settings for a long time. For decades, the public nurse, the social worker, the pediatrician, the internist, and the counselor have worked side by side. If they have not thought of themselves as a health care "team," their combined activities nonetheless resulted in that kind of work. And often, they have seen themselves as a team, held meetings and conferences together, and examined their collective process.

Health workers in public settings do not, it can reasonably be argued, need further instruction in collaborative models of care. Their need at present is an assurance that their clinics and jobs will remain open. Recent funding cuts in the public sector have jeopardized a number of very important programs, most notably those in poorer sections of the inner cities of the United States. If the politicians who control health care programs do not restore the funds they have cut, it is academic to talk about collaborative care in that sector.

If the programs do endure, however, some issues will have to be addressed. One would first have to point out that, historically, public sector medicine has been focused around the care of the poor. Models of collaborative care that have been developed in the public sector have been examined, not as ways of providing health care to the public as a whole, but rather as ways of providing less costly care to the poor. This bias has undercut the vitality and significance of many creative programs that were begun in the public sector, and it has limited the concerns of health policy planners to doing the least amount of program for the least cost in this sector. An alternative view would be to look at experiments in the public sector as creative endeavors, the significance of which can be extended to society as a whole.

Public health medicine has also had internal problems when it comes to collaborative care. It has pursued a very biomedical model of health and illness, so that psychological care has often been separated from, not integrated into, health care. Some workers in the public sector have been suspicious of counselors and therapists; others have felt it inappropriate to include therapy services in community health programs; still others have preferred to trim counseling services on economic grounds. If public health clinics are to continue, questions of collaborative care, psychological intervention, and attention to family (as well as other social and/or political) factors will need to be discussed. At base is the question, Do the poor receive the same kind of care as do those more fortunate members of our society? If the rest of medicine moves to incorporate dealing with psychosocial issues, stress management, nutrition, and exercise, will the programs serving the poor continue to exclude them on the grounds that they cost too much? (And can this even be argued, given the severe effect of psychosocial issues on the health status of the poor?)

HMOs

The fastest growing form of health care organization today is the health maintenance organization. Often structured on prepayment or capitation, these programs have been modeled after early cooperative programs such as the Health Insurance Plan (HIP) in New York, the Kaiser-Permanente Hospitals which began on the West Coast, and the Seattle's Group Health Program. The initial models were nonprofit programs. Now, most HMOs are for-profit organizations, often parts of large financial conglomerates, involved in health care on a broad nationwide basis, and applying the principles of "vertical" and "horizontal" integration of services.

The HMOs are run by businessmen, not health professionals. In spite of (or perhaps because of) this, many HMOs do try to encourage preventive health care. They discourage unnecessary surgery; they try to keep the overall costs of health care down (it is in their financial interest to do so, since every dollar spent comes out of their year-end profits). They are in a position to maximize their purchasing power, and to apportion their resources in a logical, planned way—which contrasts favorably with the virtual anarchy of the private health care system.

The type of care given in HMOs varies tremendously; so does the type of organization they follow. Depending on their particular model, they may emphasize the family physician and/or a gatekeeper concept. On the other hand, they may shun family physicians entirely, basing their organization on a panel of highly trained specialists who provide medical back-up and consultation to a large array of front-line nurse-practitioners and physician assistants—thereby turning a profit, as they save money on physician salaries. Some of them cover mental health services—but only those that seem urgent by DSM-III diagnoses. Others provide a limited, fixed amount of counseling or therapy, whatever the diagnosis. Some have on-site therapists, while others subcontract their mental health treatment to a nearby mental health facility. Some provide a great variety of ancillary services, believing that such services will save them money in the long run. Others refuse such services on the grounds that they cost too much money now, and that HMO membership is not stable because many people move about year by year, change jobs, leave the HMO, and so on. Because many different attitudes towards counseling and collaboration exist among HMOs, we can ask, What factors would incline HMOs to utilize therapy and counseling services more efficiently, in a collaborative way? How many of them see the issue of collaboration as a basic concern to investigate. How many have the capacity to take a long-term view and seek to develop the health of their clients over one, two, and three decades, not just to save money in the current fiscal year.

Other questions involve the type of service available at an HMO and who controls them. Does the physician, therapist, or administrator decide who is eligible for therapy, and for how many sessions? Does anyone receive a financial incentive for keeping therapy costs down? If so, who? Do therapists share in any savings of medical expenses engendered by the patients they treat? How much autonomy do physicians or therapists both have in the program.

Crane (1986) has opened the door on these thus-far unasked questions in an excellent critique of the therapist and the physician's position in an HMO. According to her,

> It seems that at this early stage of the game the primary care physician-family therapist team is simply not a reality for either physicians or therapists unless they have a very creative structure, a large grant, or both. Although the health maintenance organization may be an important beginning step to building this sort of team, currently the relation-

ship of the family therapist to the primary care physician within the health maintenance organization is a sort of shotgun marriage, with the two disciplines brought together . . . by the promise of a piece of the economic action and the hope of moving health care in a more family-oriented direction (p. 23).

The carrot and the stick held over the primary care physician by the health maintenance organization are in turn held over the therapist by the primary care physician. The 'carrots' of increased referrals and participation in a family systems approach to medicine are reinforced by the 'sticks' of being limited to only the authorized number of sessions and the requirement that treatment measure up to the primary care physician's standards if more referrals are to come (p. 24).

Once again, the underlying question for all collaborative care in an HMO is, what financial incentives are being provided, and under what kind of restraints and/or freedom do the psychosocially oriented personnel function.

I can envisage an HMO composed of many modular "satellite" clinics. Basic primary care would be provided at the local level by small clusters of practitioners. Perhaps there will be one or two family physicians, or a pediatrician and an internist; perhaps a nurse practitioner; most likely a primary care counselor. Other personnel could be added as needed. This small local unit would have the back-up of the HMO local community hospital, as well as access to the local panel of specialists. For problems beyond the expertise of this community-based group, patients would be referred on to the tertiary care hospital for specialists' services.

This model is especially appealling because over 95 percent of all needed health care services would be provided on site at the small local modular office. The small office could continue to function as a primary care, family-oriented practice. Patients would get to know their group of providers. The result would be very much like a series of linked family practices. In other words, family physicians, primary care counselors, and patients would all be satisfied with the range and capacity of services available at the primary care level.

I understand that some of the HMOs currently affiliated to university family medicine departments are trying to research the long-range cost savings of integrating preventive care and primary care counseling into the available panel of services. This type of work is desperately important to the future of collaborative health care.

I have not discussed the actual models of collaborative work in HMOs, because they differ so widely, and because their range really resembles what has been discussed above under the models in private practice. The main difference in the HMO model stems from the restraints put upon both medical care and counseling by the plan's administration. Instead of a two-way relationship between physicians and counselors, staff members in an HMO are involved in triangular and even more complex relationships with the administration, other staff members, and so on. The structure resembles those in other large, tertiary care, clinic and/or teaching settings.

The Role of Clinics in Academic Settings
and of Academics in Clinic Settings

A word should be said about the particular role of clinics in academic settings, and about the role of the faculty attached to academic medical and/or behavioral science departments.

Many family medicine departments are already quite collaborative. So are some other medical school departments, to varying degrees. Because much training in family medicine and other primary care fields takes place in an interdisciplinary context, its teachers as well as its trainees are inclined to accept the model of at least some collaborative care.

Many clinics in primary care training programs are run with the aid of "behavioral scientists"—counselors, social workers, therapists, students of family process, medical sociologists, and so on. Training programs both at the medical school and at the residency level utilize a good number of social scientists to teach basic notions about family dynamics, psychotherapy, normal development, emotional response to disease, and so on. Psychiatrists have long been involved in this collaborative teaching. Increasingly so, too, have been psychologists, family therapists, and social scientists. Simply having these colleagues present and accessible has meant a great deal to many young trainees; exposure to these teachers has opened doors for many to the world of psycho- and family dynamics.

Recently, some medical and nonmedical faculty members have shown interest in moving out into at least part-time private practice. There are several reasons for this:

- Staff salaries need to be supplemented;
- Faculty members feel a need to be involved in actual practice as well as in teaching;

- The collaborative care model has attracted more and more interest from those involved in teaching the psychosocial aspects of family (and primary-care) practice.

As they move into part-time practice, these faculty members accomplish a good deal, I think. They serve as role models to their students. They learn first-hand the challenges and problems involved in collaborative work and are better able to teach it to their trainees. And, finally, importantly, they become more aware of the health care financial structure, and of the constraints and guidelines of practice in "the real world." All of this cannot but help the trend towards collaborative care.

These academicians are valuable in other ways. Because they are the teachers, what they do as well as what they say influence their trainees. Because they tend to be articulate, they can popularize what they learn. And because they are connected with academic departments, they are in a position to accomplish some of the research into collaborative care that needs to be done. Although it is in the interests of the private sector—private practices, HMOs, and so on—to carry out research into the collaborative model, they may not always recognize this. The private health care sector is not known for spending lots of money on research—but, rather, in spending a lot of effort to turn a profit. They have not been inclined (until fairly recently) to start up investigative projects. But the essence of an academic department lies in its capacity to devise and carry out research while at the same time carrying out its teaching work. The interest of faculty members in collaborative practice, therefore, may be vitally important to developing the research necessary to convince others that collaborative care is efficient and practicable.

EIGHT

Starting Up

Many people ask how they can start or join a practice that provides collaborative health care. How does one go about it? There are a number of considerations that apply to almost every practice situation, while other factors are particular to private practice, clinics, HMOs, and so on. A great deal depends on just who is initiating the invitation for collaborative practice in the first place—a physician, a therapist, the directors of a health maintenance organization. The main guidelines I would offer in any situation are: move cautiously, constantly define your goals and objectives, and say whatever you feel is important.

Finding One Another:
How to Look for a Collaborative Colleague

Probably the first consideration in doing collaborative work concerns whether the practitioners are new to their work or not. Usually, collaborative work begins when one practitioner (most often, a physician) decides to take on a (psychosocially oriented) colleague in order to provide more collaborative care. This initiates a recruitment process in which one party already has a clientele practice. If both the physician and the counselor have busy practices, they will have to decide whether to join these practices together (and if so, how: loosely? tightly?), or whether one of them will have to leave where he or she is and work on the other's turf—that is, the counselor will leave his or her practice to join the physician. In any case, these structural factors are key determinants of the process.

If the practitioners are relatively inexperienced, newly trained, and without a current practice, but interested in starting collaboratively, the situation is quite different. Each colleague is starting out fresh, and they will tend to be more equal in the process.

Practitioners who are recruited into an HMO will also tend to be on relatively equal footing, in so far as they are also all new to the practice.

This consideration aside, the basic problem in starting collaborative work is how to find the right colleague. In this endeavor, nothing beats word of mouth. In every community, most health care professionals have a reputation of one kind or another—they are known to be psychosocially oriented or not, open to new ideas or not, traditional or experimental, and so on. Whoever is looking to begin a collaborative practice will do well to ask around for advice on potential coworkers. Listen to what people have to say. Then look for someone who seems to share your basic values and basic attitudes. Call people up. Visit them. See how it feels to spend some time together. Once an opportunity develops, the main factor affecting how well people are going to work together is usually their personal compatibility—in other words, how well do they fit with one another? Are their ideals, values, work ethic, and personalities compatible in the long run or not?

Therapists looking to work with one or more physicians should begin by clarifying their objectives. It is easier to begin simply by accepting referrals from some physicians, thereby getting to know them better first. If this is working out, then a move to the physician's office will not be such a huge change. One main concern should be how open the physician is to psychosocial ideas. Also, what kind of style does he or she have? How much control will the physician want over treatment overall, and does the therapist share this perspective? Disputes over physician control often severely hinder efforts at developing collaborative care.

A therapist who moves into a physician's office will want to clarify matters such as rent, fees, and the freedom to have referrals from other sources. There should also be a "safety valve" clause permitting either party to step out of the relationship after a three month period, should it not be working out. Most therapists will also want to clarify the arrangements for meeting together to discuss the patients, any other mechanisms for sharing information about patients, and how decisions will be made about any patients treated in common. Simple economic issues such as the use of the phone, payment for the services of the practice's secretaries, and arrangements for the waiting room should also be clarified beforehand.

Physicians who are looking for a counselor should also start by knowing what kind of counselor they want. Do they want a social worker skilled in working with problems of the elderly—housing, transportation, and nutrition? A nurse practitioner skilled at working with young mother and children, and at making home visits? A trained family counselor? A therapist with a Ph.D.? Would they rather have a *subordinate* colleague who will (unquestioningly) follow the protocol they put forth, or do they want a therapist who provides more mutual (give-and-take) collaboration?

If the therapist is going to be on a salary, the physician should clarify whether incentives will exist to reward greater productivity. If the practice bills for therapy services, the physician should clarify what percentage of this income is expected to revert to the therapist, and, again, what incentives exist. If the therapist is going to bill as an independent service, the physician should clarify what the therapist is supposed to pay for rent, phone, office expenses, and so on, or what percentage of the therapist's gross income goes for overhead expenses.

Once the new colleagues have decided that they share common values and a common perspective, and once they have agreed on the guidelines for their economic arrangement, they are ready to begin.

Physicians or counselors who decide to work in an HMO have other questions to ask. They need to clarify how much their salary depends on their productivity and how much on their cost-effectiveness. What are the rules governing referrals for therapy? Is there a limit to the number of sessions a patient can receive? What are the arrangements for mutual discussion? Such simple features of an HMO-type health plan define the working relationships of therapists, physicians, and the administration. If counselors pull in one direction, physicians in another, and the administration in yet a third, the staff will become dissatisfied and people's working relationships will suffer. If the HMO rewards staff for saving overall health care costs on the patients they treat, there will be an incentive for preventive work. If the HMO punishes staff for using "extra" services, there will be an incentive *not* to involve counselors and other ancillary personnel in patient care. These are subtle structural differences that have major consequences in terms of people's job satisfaction, income, and professional performance.

Potential colleagues, then, need to clarify the structural and economic issues around their working together, and they need to feel personally compatible.

Considerations of Space and Time

Most professionals want their own work space. If a therapist and a physician work for an HMO or other organization, each will want a room of his or her own. The same holds for private practice. Both counselors and physicians need their own rooms. Since it is usually the counselor who joins the physician's practice, the latter should make sure that there is adequate private and professional space for the new colleague. This goes beyond merely providing a room. It includes having space for books, files, and charts; for chairs and sofas; and for plants in the window and posters on the wall. And it includes having enough hallway space to feel unencumbered, not hemmed in; access to the bathroom, and enough waiting room space for their patients.

Since many professionals work in more than one location, it is also wise to establish clearly the hours each is expected to be in the practice. (Sometimes two therapists can share the same room, but at different times, if their hours are carefully defined.) Sharing rooms may be awkward, however, when one of the colleagues decides to spend more time in the practice but finds that no more time is available because the other person has already booked the room. A practice needs both the time and the space in which to grow.

Finally, one should be aware of the subtle feelings that accompany the sense of territory. Territory makes some people into insiders and others into outsiders and intruders. Territory imparts dominance to its owner. A therapist may feel that the practice is really the physician's, for example, because the whole thing was the physician's space first. A physician may feel like a guest or intruder when he comes for an interview in the therapist's room. Meetings between therapists and physicians sometimes work better in a neutral space, such as the hallway or kitchen, because meeting in one person's room lends that person a sense of control. Often, the sense of space can be used to counter other aspects of collaborative work. For example, in a practice where the physician tends to dominate things, conjoint therapist/physician meetings might more effectively take place in the therapist's room. Similarly, a therapist who wishes to join a somatizing family on its own terms may ask to meet the family in the physician's office first and then move on to his or her own room. Since these factors exist, they might as well be recognized and utilized.

Clarifying the Working Agreement: Communication, Decision Making

Time together is very important if colleagues are to work collaboratively. How much time they need together depends on the type of practice and the expectations of the practitioners. There are several sets of expectations at work here. First, therapist people usually expect more verbal contact with one another than physician people do. Therapists will want to talk more and at greater length about mutual patients. But second, as a rule of thumb the more collaborative a practice, the more time people will want to spend discussing common patients. The less collaborative a practice, the less people will feel a need to discuss patients in common; instead they will feel satisfied communicating ideas to one another in the chart.

When therapists and physicians work in parallel, for example, each takes charge of a different area of the patient's life. Patients are referred to the therapists for counseling around specific emotional or affective issues. The physician handles the medical problems; the therapist handles the psychosocial ones. This division can exist even though both physician and therapist have the capacity to approach problems in a contextual, systemic way. They simply agree to divide responsibility along the lines of their skill and training. This type of parallel practice, of course, may also reflect a greater split between psychosocial and biomedical issues: one or the other may be seen as primary, and their interrelationship may less often be appreciated. In this type of practice, patients will less frequently be seen to explore psychosomatic issues or to work around issues raised by physical illness. Rather, problems of the mind and body are seen as essentially separate. Practices such as this want fewer meetings between physician and therapist than do practices more involved with psycho/medical issues such as compliance, the family's involvement in a patient's illness, or the need to see and situate an illness in a systemic way. Those attracted to a more parallel practice often feel more at home with divided responsibilities. Those interested in working more closely together because they view illness and emotional factors as intertwined will want to make more decisions (about more issues) together.

We have found that it is helpful to have a regular time each week for both therapists and physicians to sit down and discuss issues involving the patients they're treating together. The time can be used to discuss other issues (hospital policy, problems with the local mental health center, conflicts with other consultants, Medicaid developments), but at least it's already *available*. When time is not regularly available, people fall out of touch, make hasty decisions about patients they are treating together, get irritated at one another (feel stepped on and bypassed) and the coordination of care is lost and irretrievably damaged.

It is important to have a way of communicating information about important recent developments with patients—a suicide attempt, a heart attack, a family crisis. In our practice, if we do not contact one another in person, we leave notes pinned to one another's work stations, bulletin board, or in-basket. If it's urgent, day or night, we will call one another by phone. Rapid exchange of information is necessary for several reasons: (1) it counteracts the patient's ability to triangulate physician and therapist, (2) it alerts colleagues to critical information that affects treatment or has developed in the course of treatment, (3) it provides for mutual decisions if basic treatment issues are involved.

We also find it helpful for everyone to write notes in the patient's chart summarizing what took place in both the medical and counseling visits—including no-shows, cancellations, emotional issues discussed, and physical complaints elicited. To this end we use a single chart for each patient (placed within a family folder), and we ask each person who has contact with the patient, receptionists included, to write in the chart.

Many disputes can arise over decision making. For example, should a patient in psychotherapy receive medications? If so, who should decide—the physician prescribing the medicine, the therapist seeing the patient, or both together? The problem can be quite intense:

Example: Amy P. was being seen by the therapist in our practice. He asked me to prescribe antidepressants for the patient. I set up a meeting with the patient and began to prescribe antidepressants. "Wait a minute," Amy P. said, "I already been on those pills. Elavil, Norpramin. I'm not depressed. What I need is something to calm me down. Like Valium."

What is the physician to do at such a time? Of course, the ideal thing would be to check back with the therapist. But what if the latter is unavailable right at that moment? It would be nice to have all three parties together at one time, but what if that is not practicable either? Choices must be made affecting patient care: How will they be made in this or that particular practice?

Sometimes we have given the main decision-making capacity to one member of the team. For example, the therapist will make major decisions about medication and other treatment issues. But even this policy can backfire:

Example: Brenda F. was being seen in counseling with her family. The physician knew that her situation was critical, and he gave the therapist the "main say" in her care. One weekend, Brenda F. phoned the physician: "I just have to go into the hospital. I can't take it any more. Too much pressure. Linda [our therapist] agrees." The physician's efforts to reach the therapist were unsuccessful. He then (resentfully) hospitalized the patient. The next day, the therapist denied having told Miss F. she "belonged" in the hospital. Instead, the therapist said the patient had manipulated the physician into getting her out of a very unpleasant confrontational home situation.

Questions around decision making can come up in the most unexpected ways. Should the therapist be part of a decision to hospitalize a family member in a family he or she is treating? What about a person whose spouse he or she is treating? What if one of the counselor's patients develops a strictly biomedical disease—that is, for example, has an acute diverticulitis attack—goes to the physician for it, and needs immediate hospitalization. Should the decision to hospitalize be a joint decision, or does one of the professionals, claiming expertise in that area of work, take charge of the treatment at that point? How much does this lend itself to somaticization as a defense? Such questions are not only intricate and subtle, they are also common! My sense is that one must have a fairly clear policy and stick with it; secondarily, it is important to insist on quick communication of any relevant data.

Money Matters

Besides matters of power and decision making, money matters create more problems than anything else. On this account, practitioners who work together should be very clear about their financial arrangements before they ever begin.

Other Issues

Most of the other issues that come up in the course of collaborative work can be dealt with usually as they arise. The main requirement for handling these issues is mutual respect: an opinion by each practitioner that his or her colleagues are well-trained and well-meaning, that each is working honestly to provide good care for the patient, and that the solution to many disagreements can be sought in differences in outlook. Often this shared perspective will enable the practitioners to clarify any disagreements, and to try to think about which of the possible courses open to them can best help the patient and his or her family.

NINE

A Sampler: Clinical Examples of Collaborative Health Care

Collaborative health care can be helpful in many situations that arise in a primary care practice. This chapter presents examples of such work from our own practice in Everett. The examples are not intended to be all-inclusive and are not ideal examples of collaborative work to be used for teaching purposes. Rather, they are simply vignettes to give a picture of some of the work that can be done.

First, however, let us look at the types of problems that collaborative work can address. Depending on the structure of a particular practice, the following problems may usefully be taken on by involving both therapist and physician in the care of the involved patient and/or family.

FOCUSING ON PREVENTIVE CARE

Screening Evaluations

All new patients can be asked to fill out a family life events stress-inventory questionnaire. If it shows that they or their family is experiencing a good deal of stress, the physician might refer the patient (and his or her family) for a session with the practice's counselor. Similarly, all new families who enroll in the practice could meet with the counselor for a routine family session, aimed at evaluating the current stage of family development, how well it is functioning, what its members' needs are, and whether any of them are experiencing serious conflict or worry, particularly that which might be expressed in physical/

somatic terms. The counselor could also assess the family's overall health (objectively), and its own view of how healthy it is (subjectively). Admittedly, such an intake screening would be costly in terms of counselor time, but if the economics of the practice were appropriate—that is, if preventive medicine were rewarded—it could be done.

A Yearly Family Health Maintenance Checkup

This type of visit would include a regular family interview with the counselor as noted above, as well as a general medical checkup for all its members, with lab tests, yearly Pap smears, and so on, as required. Such a checkup would resemble what the founders of the Peckham Experiment did. To qualify for such a yearly visit, a family would have to be registered or enrolled in the practice in toto. Because of time, money, and personnel constraints, such a plan might be used only for a few of the families in the practice. This might be on a voluntary basis, or it might be as part of a research protocol aimed at studying, say, 15 percent of the families in the practice this way, and designating another 15 percent of the practice as a matched control sample, similar families who do not receive such a yearly checkup.

Adjunctive Treatment

Many common medical situations lead to serious repercussions on the families of those involved. A family member is suddenly diagnosed as having a serious illness—cancer, diabetes. Someone suffers a grave and disabling condition—a heart attack, a stroke. A parent or grandparent dies, leaving the family in a state of grief. Physicians usually understand that such experiences are difficult for everyone involved, and they have traditionally offered to be available to those in distress, should they be needed. However, it is not routine medical practice to invite the surviving family members in for a discussion. This could be done, however, either by the therapist or by the therapist and the physician together. Such a family meeting would serve to clarify the situation, both for family members and for the health care practitioners. They could discuss the changes the new illness has forced upon them and what new resources the family might need. Such meetings can establish lines of communication that prove useful later on.

TREATMENT OF PSYCHOSOMATIC AND/OR
STRESS-RELATED ILLNESSES

The simplest benefit of having a therapist working with a primary care physician is in the management of psychosomatic stress-related disorders. I am thinking here about problems such as migraine or tension headaches, asthma, peptic ulcer disease, angina, and chronic pain. Once the patient accepts the notion that emotional or family stress is making his or her physical symptoms worse, the conjoint use of a therapist can be a real help. For example, patients can learn relaxation techniques. They can become more aware of their body's messages. They can discuss their lives and feelings with the counselor, thus identifying patterns, problems, and areas of concern that they can alter. Discussion of family issues could lead to the therapist's involving others of the family members in counseling, and in working out family tensions.

Exploring Ways Stress Affects the Body: Constant Tension

People are often unaware of how tense they are. Many chronic pains stem from muscle tension and fatigue, poor posture, or constant wear and tear on different parts of the body, combined with a lack of exercise. Constant fatigue is also a symptom of unabating strain, both physical and psychological. This problem can be explored in a health care setting if the practice's emphasis is on health, not disease, and if appropriately trained personnel are available to help patients cope with their tensions. Such a stress-modification therapist could, for example, instruct patients in controling tension through biofeedback, relaxation techniques, hypnosis, or meditation.

Coping with Anxiety and/or Depression

Other people unaware of how their bodies react to stress may experience feeling-states related to anxiety or depression, but misinterpret them as something "physical." For example, they may hyperventilate when they are anxious, but instead of identifying the resulting somatic feelings as hyperventilation/anxiety, they imagine that something is wrong with their heart, think they are about to pass out, or feel that they are going to die. Similarly, the sluggishness and deep fatigue that accompany depression may easily be mistaken for a physical illness: "Doctor, why don't I have more pep?" the patient asks. A sleep disturbance may lead to requests for stronger and stronger sleeping pills rather than to an exploration of the depression that is keeping the patient awake.

SUBSTANCE ABUSE PROBLEMS

Given the increasing problem of alcohol and other substance abuse, physicians can certainly use the skilled services of therapists to help patients cope with drug dependence and alcoholism, both in themselves and in another family member. Doherty and Baird have written especially well about ways of approaching this problem (1983), which has been estimated to affect between 15 and 45 percent of patients in any family practice.

MARITAL OR FAMILY CONFLICTS

People often suffer marital or family problems in silence. This runs the gamut from child and wife abuse to people who develop troublesome physical symptoms in a stressful family context. Often people are unable to focus all by themselves on the problems that make them suffer; instead, experiencing some physical symptom, they come to the family physician, who must recognize it for what it represents. Sometimes, of course, people bring such problems to their family physician for what they are—personal and family problems. In fact, this happens more frequently than people's initially bringing such problems to a therapist. When physicians have a counselor or therapist with them in their medical practice, though, it is much easier to help the patient and/or family get the appropriate treatment, because access to the therapist is more simply arranged.

PROBLEMS OF REPEATED PHYSICAL COMPLAINTS IN A FAMILY MEMBER WITHOUT "OBJECTIVE" FINDINGS

All physicians are familiar with patients who present themselves over and over again with unrelenting physical complaints. All physicians have had to deal with "neurotic" mothers who repeatedly bring their child(ren) to the office, complaining that they have belly pains, headaches, constant colds, earaches, unexplained fevers, and the like. And yet, whenever an explanation for the symptom is sought, no "illness" is found. In cases like these, it is helpful for the physician to have a counselor on hand to investigate the family, interpersonal, and psychodynamic contexts in which such complaints occur.

ISSUES INVOLVING COMPLIANCE

These issues almost always involve some family dynamic that is being kept a secret from the physician.

Other examples and categories can be found. The point is, however, that easy accessibility to a counselor greatly aids the primary care physician; so, in fact, does access to a medical practitioner aid the primary care therapist, who may very well wish his or her patient to get a physical exam, blood tests, and a general medical checkup, just as part of his or her overall evaluation. Being together in the same practice, in the same office, makes it easy on both counts.

The following are examples of collaborative work from our own practice:

Example 1: A lady with a heart problem and an alcoholic husband (written by Linda Atkins, M.A., Everett Family Practice).

F., age 50, is a pretty, though overweight, Italian woman who had seen Bob [Robert Singer, physician] because of obesity and eating disorder problems. She was also very depressed, apparently because of an enmeshed family system in which she played a helpless and martyred role.

During the first session she recounted many of these family problems, mostly involving her two sons and their wives. However, at the end of this session my feeling was that the real underlying problem was in her marriage relationship. She had been married nearly 25 years to S., a man with a drinking problem. Though she had on several occasions tried drastic measures, at one point even attempting a separation, she had never been able to effect any change in his drinking. She felt totally helpless and completely stuck around this issue. It was my assumption that she focused on problems in the larger family system as a way of distracting herself from this relatively hopeless situation. At the end of the session I confirmed that she had many difficult family problems, and I asked her to bring her husband with her the next time so that she might have some support in dealing with them. This was too much, too fast.

On the morning of the scheduled second appointment, F. had a heart attack. Bob and I shared the gut feeling that this was no coincidence. That feeling got reinforced when her psychologist-nephew said to her rather bluntly, "Aunt F., you chose to have a heart attack rather than face reality." She agreed with that enough to come back into therapy and stated that the hospital was the only place she felt safe.

"Safe" seemed to mean a place where she didn't have to deal with S.'s drinking.

About this time something happened in the case which, for me, pointed up the enormous benefits of working as a medical/therapist team. I was treating F. with kid gloves. She looked terrible. She was depressed, she was crying, there were dark circles around her eyes; physically, she looked like a wreck. I became very fearful that if I opened up issues too soon, she might experience another heart attack and die. At one of our regular Tuesday meetings, Bob brought up F.'s case. He was also becoming quite concerned about her, and at that point was considering rehospitalizing her. His concern was that, to leave her in the family situation might result in an emotional break-down. In discussing this, it came to light that he was fearful around her emotional state, and I was scared to death that she was going to have another heart attack. I was able to say, "I'm not concerned about F. breaking emotionally; I'm afraid she's going to die!" Then Bob was able to say to me, "I'm not worried about her heart at this point; I'm concerned about her emotional state!" We were able to have a good laugh and each of us left that meeting feeling much better. I was able to move ahead with F. in therapy in a way that would have been much more difficult without access to Bob's input. Had he been working separately as her physician, he might have put her back in the hospital without ever knowing or considering the therapeutic implications of that move.

I decided, however, not to move immediately toward the problem of S.'s drinking, but to test how F. was functioning in the larger sys-tem, what changes she could make there, and whether there were others also concerned about S.'s drinking. We started with some his-torical work. F.'s father had died when she was quite young. She was the baby in the family, with two older sisters and two older brothers. Her mother had to struggle to support the family, which meant that she was neither available for F., nor was there money for many things that F. wanted. At some point during her childhood, it became ap-parent that her brother A. was schizophrenic. She was quite frightened by some of his behavior; when he was finally hospitalized, it was a great shame to the family. She visited him regularly in the hospital, however, and he now lives with her. In an attempt to take care of her overburdened mother, F. became very adaptive and never tried to cause a problem herself. She was withdrawn, suffered terribly from eczema of her hands, and did poorly in school. She felt shame that she lacked a half-credit and had failed to graduate from high school. In talking about her early life, she stated, "I knew what I wanted, but I knew I couldn't have it." This seems to be a lesson she carried into her adult life.

Over several sessions, F. began to relate in a very different way with her family. She began to set some limits with her daughters-in-law, and she began to stand up for herself. She was quite proud of herself and began to feel better and to look better. At this point, she said she would like to bring her husband in for a session. Although it was not ostensibly set up as a session to discuss his drinking, he assumed that it was and brought it up almost immediately. It was a good session in many ways. They shared their caring for each other and discussed things not usually discussed. S. admitted that he had a drinking problem, but said he did not want to do anything about it.

Since that time, F. has stated that the only real problem she has is S.'s drinking. In a sense, this is a step forward, because for so many years she focused on outside problems to avoid this issue. However, that still leaves her in a helpless position. At this point, F. is still looking at her options. One of the things we are discussing is a family intervention, and I've consulted B. at the institute in Newton. The next step will be for me to interview F. about how much other concern there is regarding S.'s drinking. If there are enough other concerned friends and family members, then we will set up an initial meeting. That session is to educate the family/friends around alcoholism and to begin to determine one of several things: that there is not a drinking problem; that there is a problem but that F. is the only one not into protective behavior; or that there is enough concern to support a full intervention. If it appears that F. is the only one who is concerned, the therapy will then focus on her issues around that. Even if the intervention is not appropriate, F. seems to feel that once she has done everything she can, she would be able to let go and learn how to develop her own life without having to separate from S. This is where things stand now.

Example 2: The physician tells a story.

One day, in one of our regular Tuesday meetings, Linda was talking about the problem of incest. She said she'd been at her women therapists' discussion group and had heard how many, many women with somatic medical problems had a history of incest and sexual abuse. Bob listened to her for a while, then began to tell a story:

"I'd been treating this woman for fifteen months," he said. "She'd sprained her back and leg and suffered from pains in her right groin. I treated her for a sprain, and then for a chronic muscle pull, but nothing I did would make the pain go away. I'd tried heat, medication, muscle relaxants: everything. Finally, today, for some reason, when I asked her how she was doing, she answered: 'Doctor, I've been coming here for 15 months with the same pain, and nothing you've done has made it any better. I want you to tell me what's wrong.' It was like a challenge, like she was throwing down a gauntlet. I looked at her and then I said, 'Well, If nothing's made the pain any better, then it must be your nerves. You must be upset over something, and the tension is causing the pain. Do you know what might be troubling you so much?'

"She suddenly began to cry. It turned out that she'd been abused by her uncle when she was small, about five. He'd sexually penetrated her, and had hurt her. She remembers having had pains in the right groin. She could never tell anyone about it, and instead she felt bad and guilty. She withdrew from others, stayed by herself, lived a meager, hard-working, thankless life. The only person who ever seemed to understand her was her grandmother.

"Fifteen months ago the patient had an accident and developed pain in the right groin. A month later, just as she was recovering from this injury, her grandmother died. The pain persisted. She was unable to go back to work. She has been disabled ever since.

"She told me all of this, as if she had been primed to go off. Now she wants to see a therapist and talk it out.

Bob shook his head. "And I sit here wondering how I could have let 15 months pass without wondering why she wasn't getting any better, just trying one thing after another."

"But that's marvelous," Linda said. "You said just the right thing, and then she was finally able to trust you enough to tell you her secret."

"I felt there was something about the timing. . . ."

"Look," Marty said. "If we were psychoanalysts, we'd have been sitting around congratulating you on your great patience, and on your exquisite sense of timing, and on how you waited until she could tell you this herself."

Sometimes, collaborative work occurs at the interface of physician and therapist, as they discuss their own feelings, share the excitement of their interventions, and give one another permission to discover things at their own pace. For sure, the regular Tuesday sessions had helped build Bob's sixth sense to the point where he could make such an intervention.

Example 3: An elderly woman with bowel somatic fixation.

Minnie D., a 75-year-old widow, was obsessed with her bowels. She insisted on seeing me every two weeks, and spent her entire visit discussing how much diarrhea and/or constipation she had experienced, how much cramping, and what she had eaten. I spent months in an effort to control her symptoms by diet and medicine. Finally it became clear that, although Ms. D. did in fact have a chronic bowel problem, she had focused all her energy upon it, to the exclusion of the remainder of her life. I found that the "remainder" of Ms. D.'s life was actually quite lonely, empty, and bereft. Yet she refused to discuss these aspects with me, and she also refused the idea of a therapy consultation. I felt at the end of my wits.

At this point, I tried a new approach. I told Ms. D. that there was a new therapist in the practice, who knew very little about physical illnesses, but who needed to learn about them. Would she, I wondered, help me out by talking to the therapist about how her bowel problem came and went, changed from diarrhea to constipation, and left her no choice but to restrict her daily activities and worry about what her next round of symptoms would be? The patient thought about it and then accepted. She spent three sessions with the therapist, who managed in an off-handed way to get her to talk about her son, his family, her daughter who had died years ago—after which Ms. D. had had a "nervous breakdown"—her dead husband, the jobs she had held when she was younger, and the people in her apartment building. The therapist, Marty, appeared interested in her bowels, but more interested in her life. As she opened up, she seemed less depressed. She returned to my care, but was now more willing to discuss the rest of her life as well as her bowels.

I began to minimize the importance of her bouts of diarrhea and constipation. "It's all to be expected," I said, giving her a protocol of medicinal treatment for any eventuality and asking her to pin it to her wall and follow it. I tried to look bored when she talked about her bowels and interested when she talked about other things. Gradually, Ms. D. began to speak more spontaneously about her social milieu, and seemed less concerned, herself, in her bowel function. Although she continued to have an irritible bowel disorder and diverticular disease, she seemed less incapacitated, and less obsessed by it.

Example 4: A treatment failure.

Some teach by their successes. This case history tells about a treatment failure. Hopefully, one can also learn from such an example. (The narrative history follows. My comments are in a separate section afterwards, each comment keyed to the numbers in brackets.)

Mary McC. entered my practice in September, 1983, having been referred by the chiropractor down the street. In her first visit she had many complaints including bad nerves, pains in the stomach, arthritis, back pains, ulcers, gallstones, ringing in the ears, an "upside down stomach," burning in the legs, sense of having a hot face, feeling cold all over, and a past history of vaginal bleeding. She had seen a surgeon and gotten a D&C, but she stopped being his patient because there seemed little else he could do for her. She was still angry at him because he didn't have any time for her. She'd then seen the chiropractor. He had helped her arthritic pains somewhat; but, as she'd continued to have many different problems, he referred her to me for a "more thorough evaluation" [1].

Mary was 85-years-old and Irish. She lived with her husband who'd had a stroke and who was quite ill. They had no children, and she was the only person who could care for him. At our first meeting, I noted a lot of restless chatter on her part, vagueness, and anxiety. I undertook to sort out her physical and emotional problems with a full workup. At the same time, I offered to treat her "bad nerves" with a mild sedative [2]. She had already been treated with Serax 15 mg., but it was "not strong enough." Her other medications included Tagamet (for dyspepsia) and Enduronyl (for fluid accumulation).

Blood tests showed she had a low sodium, so I asked her to stop the diuretic. She did and said she felt a bit stronger. Soon afterwards, however, she phoned with severe abdominal pain. When she came in, she complained bitterly: "My nerves is all gone, my stomach feels sick, I couldn't take the Tigan, I feel depressed, I'm so weak. . . ." I prescribed vitamins and an antacid, took an EKG, which was normal, and commiserated with her over the situation with her sick husband.

Over the next few months, she complained about being tired and worrying about her husband. Mainly though she complained about upsetting bodily sensations—burning in the legs, burning in the stomach, feeling "all in," numb and cold legs, constipation, ringing in the ears. I encouraged her to talk about her situation and continued my workup, thereby uncovering "diverticulosis" and "sciatica," which I treated with medicine.

COMMENTS

[1] *The reason a patient leaves her physician often foreshadows the main problem that will arise in a new relationship. The manner, the style in which a patient leaves a physician is also highly predictive. In Mary McC.'s case, (a) she felt the surgeon didn't have enough time for her, and (b) she had been subtly "turfed" by the surgeon to the chiropracter, and from the latter (not so subtly) to me.*

[2] *She had offered "bad nerves" and "depression" as problems in her very first session. If I had pursued this right away, rather than going into an investigation of her medical condition, I might have had a better chance of short-circuiting her ensuing somatic obsessiveness.*

I prescribed the initial sedative because her agitation made me uncomfortable, and I felt she must also have been very uncomfortable. I might have done better just to acknowledge her feelings and plan to explore them with her the next time we met.

By January, 1984, we had established a pattern: Mary McC. would come in for her appointment, starting to talk before she had even gotten through the door. Once inside, she chattered nonstop, reciting one complaint after another in a monotone, giving me little time to write them all down, still less time to respond. When I tried to respond, she seemed not to hear. She wouldn't stop her talking, wouldn't acknowledge what I said, wouldn't engage me in a discussion. She'd just ramble on to another set of symptoms. When I brought this to her attention, she'd apologize perfunctorily, then continue the same behavior. I wrote in one of my notes, "Doesn't listen, just talks" [3].

She stayed on her sedative and continued her regular visits. Yet soon she "upped the ante." She asked for more frequent visits, and interspersed these requests with many phone calls, inquiring about one or another physical complaint. She also visited the Emergency Room several times. "I had to go to the Emergency Room last week," she'd say and then pour forth a torrent of obsessive rumination.

In 1984, she visited me 23 times:

January (1): She had a bad cold, aches and pains, was nervous, felt she had sinus trouble, and felt her legs were icy.

February (1): "I get that awful sick feeling now 'n' again, tired, weak, I had it bad in the back, from my head to my chin. . . ."

March (1): "Doing well, but a lot of worries about my husband. He needs a lot of attention." She still had headaches, cramps in the legs, cold feet.

April (3): [This month marked an intensification of her visits.] First visit: her abdomen ached. She thought she might have cancer. Her physical exam and blood tests were normal, but she worried she was ill with something terrible. Not sensing anything new was happening, I refilled her medicines and asked her to return in a month.

Second visit: she insisted on being seen: "I'm not feeling good. I had to come back for a visit. I'm weak, can't get out of bed." Her neck hurt, her stomach was aching, the house was cold, her knees hurt, and (finally): "Is it my heart?" I tried to talk to her about her depression, attempting to reassure her about her heart, even started her on an antidepressant.

Third visit: she came back a week later: The arthritis medicine gave her heartburn, and she refused to take the antidepressant because she feared it would make her weak. I was so dismayed that I wrote in the chart: "Patient in impossible situation: is not likely to be helped." [4]

[3] *This was already a challenge. Had I persevered, focusing on "what she was doing" rather than on what she was saying, I might have been able to help her look at her "illness behavior." By withdrawing from this attempt, I allowed her to direct our interaction, and focus it upon her somatic complaints.*

[4] *Once the physician says the patient is "not likely to be helped," a problem has developed. If the physician continues trying to help, efforts are doomed by the self-fulfilling prophecy. Furthermore, the patient will sense the lack of hope. In retrospect, it might be better to tell the patient something like, "Gee, I don't know if I can help you at this point." Or, "It must all seem pretty hopeless to you, doesn't it." The MRI people call this assuming the one-down position. It also entails telling the patient, not the chart, what I was thinking, thus taking a meta-approach to the relationship—that is, standing alongside it instead of in the middle of it. This pushes the discussion to the level on which things are "happening." Avoiding this does two things: (a) it makes treatment a charade, because no one is really convinced of its value; (b) it takes a chance away from the physician to ask the patient what she'd want to do if the situation couldn't change, thereby shifting the burden of treatment off the physician's back and offering to redefine the relationship rather than get mired in it. I did not seize this chance.*

It also raises the question of goals. Mary McC.'s goal was relief of her pains; mine was to stop her complaining. Were they the same?

May (2): No pills agree with her. She is "wobbly and weak . . . something's wrong with my heart, and the pains, and my legs, and the feet." She appeared severely agitated, and talked nonstop in a croaky voice. Both sessions were filled with constant complaining, darting from one topic to another. She would not discuss her husband now, but instead focused monomaniacally on her aches and pains. She rejected antidepressants and refused all arthritic medications. Now she started refusing to leave my office. When I rose to usher her to the door, she simply kept talking. I literally had to guide her out of the room. Frequently, she would then rush back with another question just as I was about the see my next patient [5].

At this point I raised the question of psychotherapy to her [6]. I explained that she seemed very upset, and I wondered if she might like to talk to a counselor in our office who was skilled in helping people deal with such feelings. She refused. Instead, she insisted on coming in more and more frequently with complaints of burning stomach, constipation, arthralgias, cold feet, and weakness, and wanting more frequent appointments [7].

I said I would see her every three weeks. I defined this as "supportive therapy." In spite of this she phoned more frequently, insisting on coming in every two weeks, then every week, then every few days [8].

In July she appeared with a sister who was visiting from Ireland. The sister said Mary McC. seemed in a state of exhaustion from caring for the husband yet rejected any efforts to get help. She agreed that Mary McC.'s physical complaints reflected chronic stress and exhaustion, but she felt Mary wouldn't listen to any one. "She's a worrier," she commented. "Now she thinks she has cancer" [9].

In early July, Mary McC. asked for a urine culture. In mid-July she asked for a throat culture. In late July she demanded to come in as an "emergency." She was having heartburn. She'd stopped taking her sedative. She rambled from system to system in a fervor. I tried to listen, tried to link her complaints to her worry and her exhaustion, but it was no use. She would pause for a moment, then quickly switch to complain about another part of her body. She was driving me crazy. It was all I could do to get her to stop talking long enough to get her out of the room [10]. In August she complained about her legs. She was "sick all over," distraught. I ran through one home remedy after another: oil of peppermint, charcoal, antacids, heat, rest, tea. . . . all to no avail [11].

[5] *This was another missed opportunity: As I saw this pattern develop, I might have brought her back into the office, sat her down and discussed her actions with her, commenting that she seemed to need more time, noting how upset she'd been with her previous doctor's not giving her more time, and then asking what she wanted. Instead, I was so glad when she finally left the office, I strongly resisted any thought of bringing her back for more.*

[6] *This had to be taken as a rejection, which it was.*

[7] *Mary McC. was not consciously behaving in this way. She was not deliberately trying to make my life miserable. Her behavior pointed at her problem. By reacting to her naggy behavior as others had, I missed the chance to step outside it, observe its pattern, and intervene to change it. I became part of the problem.*

[8] *Simple sympathy was not going to work. First, I was angry, not sympathetic, and she had to sense this. Second, there was no concrete basis on which I'd agree to see her "supportively," because we disagreed about what we were supposed to be doing. We each had a different agenda. We each felt jammed and cheated. This was the process that needed attention, and there was no need for superficial expressions of sympathy.*

[9] *This was possibly another self-fulfilling prophecy by someone else who'd been sucked in as part of the problem.*

[10] *In retrospect, it seems I missed a chance here to tell her how damned frustrating she was, and to explore with her why this was so. The difference in being frustrated and* saying *you feel frustrated is that in the first case the patient knows you're angry but thinks you can't talk about it, and therefore she can't talk about her part in it, either; in the second case the whole interaction is on the table to discuss,* together.

[11] *Of course.*

In late August, I again hit upon the idea of referring her to our counselor. Medicare would pay for it. I told her I felt it was important to try to talk about her worry and depression, because I felt it was her nerves that were causing so many of her bodily problems. I was at the end of my rope, and, probably sensing this, at this point she agreed [12].

She saw Martin Cohen, one of our therapists, four times in late August and September [13]. His notes comment (in part):

8/27/84 "Mary doesn't like to 'complain to anyone' about anything. She is in the middle of coming to terms with her husband's and her own mortality."

9/5/84: "Mary has a surfeit of anger and expresses only some of it directly. The rest comes out through obsessive ruminations about her health, etc. The more she tries to 'talk' to people (through complaining), the more she turns them off, and the more anger she stores up" [14].

9/21/84: "Connection between nerves, fear of her own or husband's demise, and physical pains."

9/28/84: "Pains are all worse when she is nervous. She mentioned fear of John's eventual need for a nursing home and her own physical deterioration as primary among her worries. At the end of the hour, Mary agreed that she was stressed, and that she would probably do better if she talked more about her life with someone, but she has decided to consult with Dr. Glenn (to question physical rather than psychological etiology) before making another appointment."

There were no further sessions with Dr. Cohen. After each session with him, she found her way to my office during the ensuing week with some physical complaint. After the fourth session, she came in with her same old complaints, saying "I'm not sure anything helps" [15]. Two weeks later, she (cheerily!) complained of "having those lousy old pains again—cold feet, I had to lie down, my head was heavy, I'm awful nervous; it's hard caring for John, and the health aide doesn't help."

I planned to keep seeing her every two weeks for "supportive care" [16], since I felt she needed to present her physical complaints to me and would not deal with the emotional side of things separately [17].

[12] *This was actually a good thing to do. I was making an effort to
disentangle myself from the process, since I seemed unable to cope
with it adequately. I was inviting another professional to come in and
help. The way I conceived of it, though, was not that the counselor
would help me get disentangled, but rather that he would take Mary
McC. off my hands. Because the referral was essentially riddance
behavior on my part, it was probably perceived as a rejection on Mary
McC.'s part, and was doomed thereby. The act had potential, but the
process undercut it.*

[13] *Actually, an impressive number of visits, given all that went on
before.*

[14] *This could have been something to pursue, to link up to my
own feelings about this patient. Clearly, we were both furious, but
neither of us was talking about it. I have often noticed that the patient somehow manages to create* in the physician *the very same dis-
tressing feelings from which they are suffering. We call this "mirror-
ing," and it has a rich tradition in the literature on transference and
counter-transference. The point to bringing this up is that when a
physician starts noticing feelings like this, the time is ripe for using
those feelings as a guide to understanding what's happening between
physician and patient and how that reflects the patient's basic pre-
dicament in the world.*

[15] *Rather than pick up on this invitation to discuss the "process,"
I seem to have been overwhelmed with having her back on my hands
again. I said nothing. My behavior, in retrospect, was an exact mirror
for her own. The "problem-system" had been reestablished.*

[16] *Compare comment 8.*

[17] *Here, I am unintentionally fostering a mind/body split organized around a biomedical physician and a feelings-oriented therapist.*

[18] *I wanted to get rid of her.*

*Perhaps at this point it might have worked if I'd asked her to
come in more and more frequently, or at least to phone daily. The
problem was, I felt I didn't want her to become more and more dependent on me. But I didn't really want her to be independent: I
wanted her to leave. And yet, here she was, constantly wanting to
come in. If I didn't see her, she would come or call anyway. I felt I
was in a power struggle. It was unthinkable to "paradox" her by telling her to come in more frequently, because that felt like "letting her
win." I was locked into a power struggle with her, and had to reassert
my control, rationalizing it by saying she shouldn't abuse the medical services. The better move would have been to comment on how*

Yet this plan would not work. She insisted on coming in more and more frequently. I almost had to push her out of the office to get her to leave. Finally I confronted her with this fact, but I did it so angrily that all she could do was apologize, and there was no chance of discussing "what was happening." She phoned more and more frequently, went to the Emergency Room more and more. Marty and I discussed the situation, as we had during the weeks of her therapy. I refused the idea of a joint session. I was against the idea of "paradoxing" her by demanding that she come in more and more often, or insisting on daily visits or phone calls, because—to tell the truth—I did not want her to be more dependent on the practice [18].

Mary's sister left to return to Ireland. Her neighbor, who often came in with her, told me she felt as helpless as I did. Dr. Cohen was willing to see her, but she did not want to see him. All I wanted was for her to stop annoying me: I had become like the doctor she'd left before, thereby fulfilling Martin Cohen's observation about how Mary drove people away. In spite of my training, I hadn't been unable to get beyond my anger.

Nor did I consider a consultation with a therapist. . . for myself [19]. This might actually have been reasonable, as I was locked into the situation. A therapist might have helped me get a "handle" on what was happening. Instead, I told myself this was "her" problem, not mine. If Mary insisted on bringing up physical complaints, refusing to see Dr. Cohen, refusing to take medication, and so on, and kept asking about physical illness, then I would ask for a consultation with a gastroenterologist. I then referred her to the local GI man. He of course said she was healthy, and he told her that I was doing whatever should be done. He didn't want to take her on. I instructed my secretaries not to give her any more "emergency" appointments, as they did no good. Taking the hint, Mary McC. left my practice [20].

wretched a relationship we had developed, on how angry we were at one another, and on how helpless both of us felt. Yet this did not occur to me, so involved was I in the process. I was so angry, I couldn't look at Mary McC. objectively any more.

It strikes me how I clung to the dimension of power and avoided that of affect. In a way, as Marty has pointed out to me, both Mary McC. and I were collaboratively using our power tussles to keep us both from dealing with affect—her anger at the strokes of fate, her fear of dying, her grief for her husband's situation, her guilt; my anger at her insistent clinging, my feelings around death and loss, and so on.

I was now dreading her visits. Each one seemed to be a victory for her and a defeat for me. I was by now so much a "part of the problem," I was unable to help or see that I could not help. Instead of trying to solve the problem and "cut the knot," I was myself obsessed with the power struggle. If she refused to see Dr. Cohen, then I would refuse to see her more frequently than once every two weeks. If she refused to take antidepressants, then I would refuse to take her somatic complaints seriously. Step by step, I was abandoning my commitment to provide care, which was the only basis for her coming to see me. The more ferociously she clung to the patient role—helpless, dependent, demanding—the more ferociously I refused to relinquish my doctor role—setting limits, prescribing treatment, making myself comply with her entreaty/demands. I could not get beyond this to grasp the next order of change.

[19] *This idea came from Nellie Grose from Houston.*

[20] *The circle was complete.*

AFTERWORD

Writing this up proved to be an educational experience. I was amazed at how over-involved I'd become with this patient, to the point of losing my own perspective. I was struck by Marty's correct appraisal of the situation and by my failure to take it to heart. After reflecting on this documentation, I did several things.

First, I contacted Mary McC. and asked her how she was doing. She said she was as bad as ever. I offered to see her again, and she came in. So I have another chance to help her deal with her unhappiness and somatic distress.

Next, I talked to Martin Cohen about our own interaction. I felt he had seen the problem clearly, but hadn't been able to confront me about my own behavior. We discussed this. He said some of his hesitation came from feeling like a newcomer working in "my" practice. Some came from his feelings about doctors being on a pedestal. Some had to do with his feelings about his father (whom I reminded him of) and also to difficulties he had in confronting people.

This discussion led to a critique about how we were working together collaboratively. Collaboration is not always rosy; it also opens each of us up to criticism. We have to be ready to deal with this. In Marty's case, he had to be ready to stand up to a physician 15 years older than him. In my case, I had to be open to exploring my own counter-transferential issues.

It was clear that my failure to listen to Marty was related to feelings of control and dependency, and to the use of the power dimension to cover over affective experience. This pattern had antecedents in other attitudes I had. Our discussion led us to redefine our working relationship, open it up to mutual criticism, and relabel such criticism as a valuable communication.

A final follow-up is available now. Mary's husband grew worse. She again came to the office with repeated somatic complaints. I felt there was simply nothing further I could do, and I advised nursing home care and spoke to several members of her family about this. Mary refused, however, and they could not convince her. Now she began to demand admission to the hospital for her pains. I refused. I said that she needed chronic care, seemed unable to manage on her own, and I said the hospital was not an appropriate place for her. After coming into the office unannounced, demanding to be admitted for "the burning in my side, these pains, trouble walking, all the time," she left the practice again. She went to the Emergency Room and presented herself in a state of collapse. The E.R. physician admitted her, but she asked to be under the care of another physician. After being hospitalized for several weeks and a negative workup, she was finally sent to one of the local nursing homes, a disposition which she accepted with no complaints.

Example 5: A young man's grief.

Carl J. was a 16-year-old schoolboy whose family had been in our practice for decades. He suddenly began behaving oddly, and his family was concerned. When I talked to him, he seemed preoccupied. He didn't know what was bothering him. The family thought he might be on drugs. I wondered if he was upset over something in school, problems with a girl friend, or in some kind of developmental crisis. He insisted he just didn't feel right, but had no idea what was bothering him. I asked him to talk to Linda to help figure out what was wrong.

After two sessions, Linda felt she had an answer. Carl was extremely close to his grandfather. The gentleman had died eight months earlier, and no one else in Carl's family seemed capable of taking his place and showing Carl that same degree of attachment and concern. Carl had become increasingly moody and depressed; he turned inward. He'd begun having physical complaints and doubts about himself as a person. As he talked to Linda about the problem, his grief rose to the surface, and she was able to help him express the feelings that he had for his grandfather, feelings which his undemonstrative family had not been able to help him express earlier. As his grieving occurred, his symptomatic behavior quieted down, and he seemed better, both to himself and to his family.

Example 6: The patient outflanks both the therapist and the physician.

Sally P. was a 45-year-old woman with hypertension. Her daughter Sue had been in therapy with Linda for six months for various and shifting somatic complaints, which Linda felt were related to an overly close mother-daughter relationship. For example, mother and daughter slept in the same bed, even though the daugher was 20 years old. Sally's husband Matt was an alcoholic, who would not stop his drinking. Family therapy had been suggested to them, but everyone had refused it. After a few months of therapy, Sue moved out and seemed to get better, but then Sally developed multiple somatic complaints—tightness in her chest, headaches, palpitations. She was afraid she had a heart condition.

I felt her symptoms were the expression of nervous tension. I asked if she'd see Linda on her own, and she said she would; and both Linda and I agreed on the nature of her problem. Sally insisted however on coming in (increasingly often) in a very anxious state. She would obsess over her physical worries and ask repeatedly about her heart. When I asked about her family life, she complained that I wasn't taking her physical problem seriously. So I examined her carefully. Her blood pressure was well-controled. Her EKG was unremarkable. I even arranged for her to have a stress test, and this too was normal. But her pains persisted, and she insisted they were from her heart. She worried that she might have heart trouble, perhaps even cancer. She was extremely reluctant to accept the notion that her pains might be linked to family factors, such as her husband's increased drinking.

She insisted on seeing a cardiologist, so I referred her to one. He gave her medications for angina pectoris and told her she could have angina even with a normal stress test. He said if she didn't get better she might need a cardiac catheterization. She said she was desperately afraid of having that (she might die!), but she said, if it came to that, she was ready. After I had spent a session dealing with her chest pains and referring her to the specialist, Sally complained to the receptionist that I hadn't "spent enough time" with her. This made me feel furious, because I thought I'd spent more time with her than with most patients, and had focused the whole encounter around *her* insistent physical complaints.

Sally was still seeing Linda. So Linda and I talked. Neither of us felt that Sally should have the catheterization, and both of us had told that to Sally; I predicted that Sally was going to have the procedure done, and soon.

Within a week, Sally had gone to the Emergency Room with chest pain. She'd asked the doctor there to call the cardiologist, and he admitted her for telemetric cardiac monitoring. Her pains persisted. Tests were normal. She transferred into a tertiary care center in town for cardiac catheterization, the results of which were normal.

Now Sally feels she does indeed have to be careful, because she has angina, and she is on a number of different medications to control the pain. Linda and I feel she has constructed her own reality, with the cooperation of the cardiology consultant (who, after all, acted in a totally understandable way).

Sometimes, patients escape the good intentions of both physician and therapist, develop their own view of what ails them, and deal with the perceived problem their own way.

Other examples of collaborative work could also be given, if we had the space—a family whose eight-year-old son had constant belly pains; a very anxious young mother; an anorexic teenager whose mother appeared severely depressed; a young man who had trouble concentrating. The list of treatment opportunities is extensive. Most readers can add several similar possibilities on their own.

TEN

Problems in Collaboration

Discussions by Eliot Freidson (1970) and other social scientists (compare especially Szasz and Hollander, 1956) about the conflict inherent in the doctor-patient relationship appeared to shock many patients and physicians. The myth of the cozy "complementary" relationship described by Talcott Parsons (1951), in which the patient accepts the physician as a benevolent expert and agrees to follow his or her advice and directives, does not always work. Wherever differences of social class, culture, race, sex, and age exist between patient and physician, different values and different hierarchies exist, too. The two parties often possess conflictual agendas, and scuffles for power frequently arise. The same argument holds for differences between different providers of care in a collaborative health endeavor, for relationships between these colleagues can be conflictual as well as collegial. The main conflicts that emerge involve turf and money, authority and power.

Competition is, after all, part of natural social existence. Throughout the animal kingdom, its aggressive thrust is linked to the instinct of protecting one's basic territory: creatures safeguard themselves, their kin, their turf. Human beings, however, are supposed to be a more highly evolved animal form; our social survival depends on our following mutual rules of behavior, as well as on our intelligence, instincts, and strength. The compromises civilization insists on are necessary for social development. We relinquish the freedom to act on our most primitive feelings in exchange for a place in society (protected as well as chastened by its laws). To live together, we have learned to cooperate, not bludgeon one another out of greed or anger, steal each other's sexual partners, gobble up each other's food, or shoulder others aside and take their goods. We may even do without life's pleasures if having them means that others must suffer. If others are less fortunate than we are, we treat them with respect and compassion: heal the sick and care for the poor, for we never know when we might be unfortunate ourselves.

That's how it's supposed to be. But human society can make the jungle look like a garden club by comparison. Competitiveness, greed, and cruelty are all constant and—one might even hazard—ascendant. How then will the advocates of cooperation transform their ideals into reality? This is a critical issue for contemporary America. In the health care field, as economic pressures tighten, competition among health care providers has increased. The existing incentives do not push people toward greater collaboration, but instead reward greater and greater fragmentation of care. The pie shrinks, and the (civilized) professionals scrap for their share.

Collaboration is not easy to accomplish. It takes tremendous, disciplined effort and consistent dedication. It also demands attention to the conflicts that develop at every turn.

We can group these problems into two main categories: *extrinsic* and *intrinsic*. The first group includes problems the origins of which stem from outside of the health care group. The second group includes those which result from internal factors, such as team friction, coworkers' loyalties to different disciplines, different views of the "same" problem, rivalries, jealousies, inequities in pay or time worked. The extrinsic problems are most basic, for they involve the fundamental matters of having a job, being paid, and having job security. Once these problems are settled, however, a host of intrinsic problems appear. These may sometimes be interpreted as individual (personality) problems: problems of adjustment, problems of belonging, problems of style. But this is not the truth. These intrinsic problems usually reflect some *structural* difference—for example, what rules govern people's roles, expected behavior, and protocols of their work together? What guidelines govern the team's behavior, and who makes them? Who has power to make final decisions for the group; who gets paid what; what happens when people disagree? What economic realities support the differences in influence and power?

THE BASIC ISSUES ARE ECONOMIC

The basic issues underlying collaborative health care are economic: Who is picking up the tab, thus enabling the collaborating professionals to go ahead with their work? This includes extrinsic factors such as the types of reimbursement schemes set up by the federal government, the state, and various insurance companies, as well as the licensing laws that affect any given group. One must look at the economic structure of any practice, especially the salary differences and the economic incentives. The way dollars are divided is an intrinsic factor that structures people's roles.

EXTRINSIC FACTORS AFFECTING COLLABORATIVE HEALTH CARE

The main extrinsic factor that affects the development of collaborative health care at the present time is the various state and federal laws governing reimbursement. Briefly put, all psychosocial aspects of health care receive low priority. Physicians receive less for time spent talking to patients than for doing procedures. Therapists frequently have difficulty billing Medicaid or Medicare patients for therapy services in the private setting; and groups that offer prepaid care often eliminate or restrict therapy or counseling services, thinking thereby to save money. Private insurance plans restrict access to psychotherapy. In addition, licensing laws have created obstacles for many therapists, preventing them from billing third parties for their services. The concern with cutting medical costs has led to pressures for providing therapy services only in cases where "major" psychiatric disorders exist—but this creates serious problems for therapists who deal with family adjustment crises, situational stress problems, and characterological (substance abuse, and other such) issues. Furthermore, many patients who will accept psychotherapy for a "situational problem" will not agree to have their diagnosis listed as "obsessional neurosis" or "schizophrenia" just so their insurance companies will pay for therapy; issues of privacy and confidentiality are also involved. A final complicating factor is, that insurance company codes and the DSM-III lack categories to deal with family-wide issues; they focus mainly on individual diagnoses, a (retrograde) trend that trails the level of sophistication of the therapy fields.

These and other economic factors can discourage physicians and therapists from working together. They bolster fragmentation of care and reinforce the guild mentality. Especially now with the resurgence of the biomedical model, the existence of strong material incentives for fragmented care are a major roadblock to collaborative health care. This is a problem that can only be changed by a complete reorganization of the health care systems, its nosology, its fee structure, and its modes of practice.

FACTORS INHERENT IN DIFFERENT TYPES OF PRACTICES

Depending on the type of practice under consideration, different structural factors operate to condition and/or qualify the possibilities for collaborative health care.

Traditional Fee-for-Service Practice

Traditional fee-for-service payment is still the model for most private practice. Physicians, therapists, nurses, and other professionals are assumed to be well-trained. Because of this, they are given the freedom to decide how to care for their patients, and they are reimbursed for their services. Collaborative care in the private sector is relatively younger than collaborative care in clinics, tertiary care centers, and training programs. It has also been more difficult for a variety of reasons, most notably in recent years because of the economic difficulties of finding reimbursement for the associated therapist; but there are other problems as well:

First, there are reimbursement issues for the therapist/counselor: being paid by the insurance companies, Medicare, and Medicaid for their work.

There are issues of "time," especially for the physician: The physician in private practice is reimbursed for direct service time, not for time spent sitting in with the counselor or for case-management discussions.

There are problems in conflicting outlook: therapists and physicians have different training, different perspectives on the patient's problem, different mind-sets in general, and different priorities, based upon their actual daily routine. These involve conflicts in professionally linked style and conflicts in thinking, that is, the way problems are framed (compare Bassoff, 1983 and Glenn et al., 1984). (For example, the physician who sees 750 patient visits a month may have a mind-set that does not incline him or her to initiate a discussion about one patient he has referred to the therapist. The therapist, who may be seeing 20 to 30 different people throughout the month, will be more inclined to initiate discussion about a patient with whom he is spending more time and whom he is getting to know more intimately than has the family physician. After all, it was for this that the referral was made in the first place.)

If professional practitioners decide to work collaboratively together in a private setting, certain questions will come up around their organizational structure, as well as around each professional's fees and/or salary:

First, who has taken whom into practice? Is the physician bringing a counselor aboard his or her own ship? Are two professionals deciding to start a practice together? Who has made this decision?

Second, what particular kind of therapist or counselor is entering the practice? A social worker? A family therapist? A counselor? What skills must these people have? What training? What will the patients call them? Is their work reimbursable by the insurance companies the physician accepts? At what rates? If not, how will they be paid?

Will the therapist/counselors work as free agents, accepting referrals from the physician with whom they work, but also from other interested physicians? Or will they be on salary from the physicians' practice? Will this mean they have to see a certain number of people to obtain that salary? If they see more, do they get a bonus? If fewer, are they docked? Do they give any free care (that is, care that cannot be reimbursed) as part of their job contract, letting their physician-employer swallow the difference?

How do the therapist/counselors' salaries compare with the physicians'? Do therapists have to kick back a percentage to the physician for referrals? Must they pay for office expenses?

Under fee-for-service, more procedures means more money for the physician—or other provider. The financial incentives all lie in seeing patients (specifically, those with coverage) and treating them exhaustively. Patients without coverage are financially bad for the practice, and some physicians even try to keep them at an arm's distance from the practice. (Professional medical management consultants are full of ideas for building up the number of insured patients in one's practice and scraping away the "troublesome" ones—those without coverage, or on welfare.)

Another issue concerning reimbursement focuses around eligibility for reimbursement. Just what providers will third-party payers pay; and for what services? For example, in Massachusetts, Medicaid will pay for a routine physician's visit. But they will pay a private clinical psychologist only for psychological testing. They will not pay a private social worker or psychologist for psychotherapy. If, however, the social worker or psychologist is employed in an approved mental health center, their services will be reimbursable. What happens, for example, when a physician can be reimbursed by Medicaid for seeing a patient, but a psychotherapist in the same practice cannot be reimbursed for therapy. Will the patient have to go elsewhere, to a mental health center charging twice as much as the private therapist? Pay for their own care? Settle for no care?

Market incentives encourage private practitioners to treat people with the means to pay and to see them as often as needed. If they cannot be reimbursed, therapists and other counselors in a private practice setting must either work on salary—let the practice bill for their services—or only see insured patients or those with an ability to pay.

HMOs

Incentives in HMOs work in the opposite way to those in private practice. HMOs get their money up front from the start: a lump sum at the start of the year. But the HMO must then dispense fees for all its member services. Should the money run out, the HMO is still liable for bills, and it may have to default on its own payments. If the HMO is run by a corporation, losses in one site may be covered by profits somewhere else. If an HMO is locally controled, and run, say, by the local practitioners themselves (as a PPO), the practitioners themselves may be at risk for the losses. Should there be a savings of money, of course, any or all of the HMO providers may share in it.

Financial incentives in an HMO act to discourage medical care visits. Since the HMO has its money at the start of the fiscal year, it only stands to lose money as patients come for treatment—that is, the more the HMO does for its patients, the more it can erode its own profits. Incentives reward *undertreating* by HMOs, a fact that is now (1986) beginning to arouse a considerable amount of interest and concern.

Should the HMO decide, however, that certain procedures or services are likely to benefit its patients' overall health—and thereby lower overall costs—it can arrange for these procedures or services to be provided to more and more of its clientele. Thus it will encourage modest preventive health measures—seat belts, diet training, no smoking, stress reduction—which can be shown to produce significant savings for the HMO, as well as to lead to better health for its patients, further down the road. Such an argument can be used to justify spending whatever small amounts of money are needed for preventive treatment.

Readers of this book will undoubtedly feel the same case can be— and has been—made regarding access to psychotherapy. Since many illnesses appear and/or worsen with stress, and since stress is ubiquitous, and since therapy intervention can be extraordinarily helpful in focusing on problems, diminishing stress, and resolving disputes and conflicts, one can make a simple rationale for including basic mental health services in an HMO. Such was what the Kaiser Permanente Hospital, in California did (compare Follette and Cummings, 1967; Cummings, 1977).

Kaiser offered therapy as an included benefit to its members. It found that when up to six therapy sessions were offered within the plan, overall health care costs for the population covered went down. They further found that when unlimited therapy was offered, the overall costs went down even further. Their studies have been replicated with similar results in Great Britain and the Netherlands. The lessons of this appear, however, to have been lost on many of the HMOs in the United States today. They have usually opted for either limiting or farming out their mental health services, not integrating them into the overall health maintenance plan.

Community Health Centers

The budgets of community health centers, like HMOs, permit them to allocate their resources where they feel they are needed. Thus, they could employ substance abuse counselors, specialists in adolescent medicine, social workers familiar with the problems of the elderly, and so on. The problems historically with community health centers have been (1) they typically serve a poor clientele, (2) their budgets rely on outside funding and frequently suffer from cutbacks, and (3) their professional staff frequently turns over, thus leaving the patients without continuity of care.

In the 1960s there was a vast movement toward such health centers, which attracted many dedicated health workers from a diversity of disciplines. The idealism and community commitment behind such efforts have more recently flagged somewhat, and funds have dried up. The remaining clinics are often forced to focus on the most-needed medical resources—lead testing, pediatric care, immunizations, alcoholism, hypertension, and so on—and have not been as able to offer a farther-reaching therapeutic menu. The effects of the return to strict biomedical thought have compartmentalized the problems of the usual community health center populace, making them once again trudge the rounds from agency to agency, clinic to clinic, and there has been little effort to organize comprehensive care in community clinics since the mid-1970s. Certain pilot programs affiliated with progressive-minded medical schools—Montefiore, New Haven, Rochester, Stanford—have kept this tradition alive, but today it is in decline.

The rationale advanced for dealing with the economic problems of collaborative care in HMOs holds just as well for the community health centers. Collaborative care thrived two decades ago in just such centers, and should be able to do so again, if the interest and drive were to arise again.

EXAMPLES OF CONFLICT IN A DISCIPLINE: FAMILY MEDICINE

In spite of the attempts to work together, conflicts do arise among persons, organizations, and disciplines. One example of how collaboration helped develop a field that is now undergoing a struggle to preserve such collaboration is the case of family medicine.

Over the past ten years, therapists and other systems thinkers have expended a tremendous amount of effort to help build the field of family medicine. They have taught family dynamics to family physicians, especially residents, and they have consistently raised the question: How can family physicians meet their patients' psychosocial needs? Frequently family physicians have been encouraged to learn basic counseling and referral skills. Throughout this time the family-oriented folks have had to fight uphill battles, first to establish and then to maintain their position. Initially, they were outsiders, brought into the field out of necessity. Then they were seen as apostles of an alien ideology, "the family in family medicine," who actually had the nerve to claim to represent the heart and uniqueness of the discipline they had helped found. Disputes then arose about the "real" differences between family practice and older general practice. Finally, as family medicine has at last found acceptance at the dinner table of organized medicine, the family-oriented sector has had to deal with the growing conservatism of their erstwhile medical colleagues, who now seem willing to bargain both them and their ideology away, in exchange for a mess of pottage, grants, and the chance to hobnob in fancy circles.

The main thrust of this wing of family medicine's writings seems to be to encourage family physicians to learn how to work with the family. "Working with the family" (Christie-Seely, 1984) has been presented as a skill family physicians can learn, not quite so technical or difficult as family therapy. Christie-Seely always makes a reassuring distinction between "working with the families" and "family therapy," and argues that the former lies well within the realm of family medicine. Doherty and Baird (1983) encourage family physicians to learn "primary care counselling skills," but they feel—as does Christie-Seely—that physicians should refer patients to a friendly therapist when problems become too difficult. Some of the exhortation for family physicians to learn counseling skills goes back to Michael Balint's instructions to British GPs about working at a "deeper level" with their patients (1957), and reflects an interest in psychological process that has marked family medicine since its inception.

Challenging as this approach may be, it now seems it has served to attract a few brave family medicine souls to therapy training, to create thereby a handful of curious hybrids, to cull forth a number of fascinating insights, and to frighten most family physicians away from working with families altogether! It may also have encouraged some physicians to claim (arrogantly) that they have now learned about family dynamics and can replace the behaviorists in family medicine departments. Such appropriation of collegial territory is not only petty and selfish—coupled with the economic squeeze in some departments of family medicine, whose necessities have been resolved by canning the "softer" therapy and social science folks, it transcends offensive style and approaches opportunism. In addition, it threatens to water down the complexity of family therapy exactly when therapy's sophisticated understanding is most needed to prevent cookbook, shallow work with families. Some therapists may well be saying, "With friends like these, who needs enemies?"

The main hazard of therapists' creating counseling handbooks for family physicians is not their watering down their own theory, but their being instruments of their own demise. As family medicine departments cope with financial pressures, the place of those collaborating social workers and psychologists is jeopardized. If they are eased out of some departments, then the model-in-training of collaborative care will fade, and it will be even more difficult to engage family physicians in collaborative work once they leave residency training.

INTRINSIC CONFLICTS IN COLLABORATIVE CARE

Moving from the macro- to the micro-level, one encounters conflicts that are basically intrinsic to the process of collaboration:

• Who's in charge? This covers key issues such as: Who initiates the referral? Who makes the rules for treatment? Who owns the office space? Who makes decisions about medications? Who has the last word when there is disagreement?

• What level of training have the physicians and therapist attained in their work? Are they compatible? Is there a basis for mutual respect?

• What are the practitioners' daily schedules like? How many hours do they put in? How are they reimbursed for this effort, and what is their difference in income? How do they feel about this difference?

• How are referrals actually made? Does the physician refer almost all the patients, or is the therapist/counselor given some autonomy in the process?

• What philosophy of care do the practitioners follow? Is it compatible?

• How much discussion takes place between physician and therapist?

• How are decisions made?

Earlier, we examined social work's contribution to the developing idea and the burgeoning practice of collaborative health care, focusing on its involvement in several sentinal practices in which social workers joined family (primary care) medical practices. In this section, I want to focus on the social work critique of such collaborative efforts. This critique is a *friendly* critique, a critique "from within." The social work analysis of efforts at collaborative care comes from a perspective of wanting such efforts to succeed, of learning from shortcomings in order to strengthen future efforts. This analysis is not aimed, as some others are, at dismissing the model as unrealistic, overly costly, crackpot, or politically repugnant. This makes the social work critique even more poignant, for by and large it has been raised only to be ignored by others engaged in this "mutual" effort, just as social workers themselves have had to fight for access to patients in medical settings and for respect from their potential colleagues.

The further development of collaborative health care does not depend on sweet idealism or on the simple desire to work together that spurs different health professionals to "try it out." Rather it depends on the existence of sound material incentives for such practice and on the reorganization of services where necessary. To accomplish this, we need a penetrating understanding of the collaborative process itself.

Critiques of collaborative efforts have often appeared in the social work literature—especially the journal *Social Work in Health Care*—for the past 10 to 15 years. Articles have discussed tensions between team members, territorial disputes, differences of style and perspective, as well, increasingly, as differences revealed through analysis of structural (not just ideological) differences. For example:

A pioneering discussion of the strains among health care professionals trying to work together is Banta and Fox's piece "Role strains of a health care team in a poverty community" (1972).

Gilchrist and coworkers (1978) evaluated a number of collaborative efforts between social workers and physicians. They found that the main difficulties were insufficient preparation for the scheme, poor communication between general practitioners and social workers, and the inadequate provision of facilities for social workers on the practice premises. Two-thirds of their respondants described their experience as rewarding.

Lowe and Herranen (1978) have described a series of stages in the collaborative process through which health care professionals can be expected to pass as they attempt to develop a more interdisciplinary collaborative practice.

Dana, perhaps the foremost writer in the United States on the collaborative process, has (with Banta and Deuschle [1974]) summarized many of the pros and problems in such work, in "An agenda for the future of interprofessionalism," and "The collaborative process" (1983). As an educator, she, like others who propose collaborative models of health care, considers the years of one's professional education as the critical place to start developing a sense of working together.

Bassoff, in a blistering critique of the notion of collaborative care, questions whether such care can in fact succeed, especially in the private practice sector. She points out that physicians continue to control access to care. Through their referral power and through their customary position as the leader of the health care team, physicians function as gatekeepers, deciding who gets referred to the social worker and who does not. In spite of all the work done around the concept of the health team, physicians continue to view social workers, nurses, and other colleagues as "extenders" of care, as people whose role is to augment the physician's role (Bassoff, in Miller, 1983; also citing Kindig). Furthermore, today the matter of including social workers and others into the health care team increasingly focuses on whether they can pull their own weight—that is, on whether their services are reimbursable, on whether they can draw in needed funds, and on whether money spent on their salaries can lead to greater cost savings in the future.

Bassoff suggests that relationships among the different health care providers have not substantially changed over the past decade. In fact, she feels that it is less acceptable now to discuss conflicts and differences because of increasing competition for the health care (and counseling) dollar. Yet, while the concept of health care has finally expanded to include various psychosocial factors, Bassoff notes that the new psychosocially oriented members of the health care team have actually given tacit support to the growing "medicalization" of social problems. By joining their work to that of the physician, they have come increasingly under the power of the physicians' persistently biomedical world. What are the social workers and other counselors getting? What are they giving up? Bassoff suggests that they are in danger of losing the values and unique perspective of their own discipline, which does not go along with the search for greater profits, and which often views the social and economic aspects of human problems.

But there are other problems besides physician dominance. Increased competition between the fields of nursing and social work has led to turf disputes. The emergence of newer and newer counseling professionals, marked by disputes over access to third-party payments, has led to great competition in the realm of counseling and therapy.

> In California, the scenario is striking, almost comic, in the elbowing which exists in the therapy marketplace among psychiatrists, psychologists, and [other] experts. The unanticipated consequences of licensing has made the social worker an entrepreneur, creating incredible new income sources for the sale of continuing education credits. The brochures arrive daily. Everyone carries a calling card. Like medicine and law, there is little pretense to monitor quality of practice, which licensing had promised. In hospital settings, new partners like health educators, patient representatives, home health specialists, grief counselors, and others vie for recognition. Who delivers what we refer to as psychosocial services in any setting is entirely dependent upon the politics of who got there first, and who can create third-party payment income (Bassoff, 1983, pp. 124-125).

Bassoff's suggestions fall in the category of professionals learning respect for one another:

1. Students of health disciplines must learn to *appreciate* the skills, knowledge, and expertise held by other providers, in order to respect and value one another's input in the decision making of the health team;

2. Students of health disciplines must learn the *functional roles* of providers within the team;

3. Students of health disciplines must develop the *interpersonal skills* necessary for practice in a multidisciplinary health team; and

4. Students of health disciplines must learn the *skills of group behavior* such as leadership, conflict resolution, and negotiation, based on the obvious fact that the team, no matter how loosely constructed, is a group of people who need to work together.

HUNTINGTON'S CONTRIBUTION:
COLLABORATION OR CONFLICT

Several voices have been raised to analyze collaborative health care. But perhaps the most penetrating analysis of interprofessional conflict appears in June Huntington's excellent study, *Social Work and General Medical Practice: Collaboration or Conflict?* The author, a medical sociologist, began her study with the assumption that social work and general medicine are such different fields that they possess two different cultures. An understanding of the differences, she hoped, would help practitioners understand the source and significance of the conflicts that arise when they try to work together. While Huntington deals only with social work and medicine, hers is a generic critique of the problems inherent in all collaborative efforts in health care, whether they involve nursing, social work, medicine, or family therapy. (For the time being, let me group all therapists and counselors together, even though there are myriad conflicts between therapists of varying stripes and persuasions, between counselors of different degree, and between adherents of different schools and different approaches. Whatever we find in our analysis of differences between physicians and social workers can be applied to any of the other groupings.)

Huntington begins by distinguishing between *structural* and *cultural* differences between professions. The former include the kind of data one finds on epidemiological, statistical examination of the fields; the latter, data which relate to their ideas, values and beliefs.

Structural differences between medicine and social work include such items as the following: Medicine is an older profession than social work, with a long history of importance and acceptance. Its practitioners tend to be older than social workers, middle-aged and beyond, whereas social workers are often in their twenties and thirties. These factors reinforce medical dominance in collaborative work; younger, more independent-minded social workers will find it difficult to confront older GPs on issues of conflict.

Many social workers are women, often unmarried, whereas physicians tend to be men with families. Huntington suggests this sexual difference is the most important factor in promoting medical dominance, as it recreates male-female, father-daughter, husband-wife, dominance-submission type relationships in many efforts at collaborative care. More needs to be known about interaction between other groups of physicians and social workers—such as women physicians and women social workers, and so on.

Physicians also tend to come from a better-situated class than do social workers. Their training is longer and more extensive, and they make a good deal more money than social workers, both of which are factors that reinforce their dominant position. In addition, their work is usually individual, working alone or in small associations. Fee-for-service tends to be piecemeal work, making physicians into small entrepreneurs, emphasizing their individuality and the aspect of personal control over their own lives and finances—both of which are alien to most social workers. This also helps explain physicians' possessive treatment of their patients: The patients are their actual source of income. Physicians are usually their own bosses, whereas social workers are usually on some kind of salary.

Furthermore, social workers often work with a less-advantaged clientele in general than do physicians, which gives them lower prestige in society's eye. Most family physicians draw their referrals from the lay culture. Few social workers attract patients by self-referral. Instead, they see clients in institutional settings, or on the referral of others. These differences lead to a different sense of prestige.

These and other structural differences lead to different cultural norms and values, such as regards the meaning of time, the sense of change, the task of one's occupation, and the view of prevailing social customs.

Huntington's is an excellent beginning in the analysis of professional differences. I would not argue with its basic conclusions. Instead I would ask, what will be the result of the changes in occupational structure that are now happening:

- More women are going into medicine;
- Men are going into social work and nursing;
- More physicians are working on salary, many of them with little control over their livelihood;
- More social workers are moving into private practice counseling and therapy;
- Reimbursement for services by social workers has evolved but still varies greatly from state to state in the United States.

The stereotypic cliche of "the family physician" and "the social worker" are actually changing now, and that is itself one of the main factors leading to stress in working together—for there are trends in both professions today that would like to expand the proper scope of their work into areas long ago claimed by the other (or related) health care disciplines. Professional role and identity are shifting, along with the demographics of the professions themselves. The resultant indecision has led to increased conflict among colleagues. A psychosocially oriented physician may have more in common with a psychosocially oriented psychotherapist, when it comes to many issues involving patient care, than he or she has with the physician down the street. A young female family physician may have more in common with the young female social worker than she does with the (male) family physician who was her mentor. At the same time, professional stickiness is hard to overcome, when the chips are down and the etiquette of physicians' (as well as other professionals') sticking together may undermine many efforts to resolve interprofessional difficulties in working together.

But to return to Huntington's book, she then moves from the structural differences to the cultural ones. Under this rubric she considers such topics as the mission, aims, and tasks an occupation sets for itself; its focus and orientation; its epistemology and sense of what constitutes "knowledge"; its sense of technology and technique; its language; its ideology; its identity; its status and prestige. Similar aims between medicine and social work lay the basis for competition over turf and overlapping of work. Differences in focus and orientation may lay the groundwork for disputes about the nature of the real problem. Differences in the degree of action-orientation are linked to the sense of time and change, and can lead to disputes over how quickly physician or social worker should try to change a patient or the patient's family.

Huntington then draws a picture of the two professions as they existed in the mid-1970s. In her analysis, medicine still follows the strictures of the biomedical model; it is concerned with the identification and treatment of disease. Physicians, often working on their own in solo or group office-based practice, may feel that time is money. They tend to be action-oriented, and are jealous of how they spend their hours, certainly being loath to spend much time in discussions unless the time is somehow reimbursable. Physicians also tend to look down on all other health professions and feel they are authorities on virtually everything. At the same time, they can be extremely defensive about their position, especially insofar as they are aware that they are legally responsible for the patient's care.

Social work by contrast tends to follow the biopsychosocial model. The field is concerned more with psychosocial problems, with the social and political dimensions of care, with community, and with process. It has a long tradition of identifying itself as the caretaker of the less-advantaged in society and often tends to see people as innately good, but trapped in a matrix of social forces beyond their control. Social workers also tend to be less individualistic, more oriented toward collective work. They have a better sense of group dynamics and of the potential role of community factors. Whereas physicians are more action-oriented, social workers tend to be more comfortable with listening. I would wonder how much these differences are really expressions of a possible male/female difference, for this and several other differences between the two occupations certainly appear to echo sex-role differences. (I would, for example, wonder what impact the presence of more women physicians will have on this phenomenon.) Each occupation has its own language, its own terms. Each is, Huntington points out, undergoing an identity crisis: Some social workers are moving toward greater autonomy and into the private sector; some physicians, especially those in primary care and family practice, are looking to a more comprehensive approach in their own work.

She then discusses major differences in ways the two occupations relate to their patients or clients. The social worker "accept[s] and sometimes idealise[s]" the patient. General practitioners have a "profound ambivalence" toward their patients. Family physicians often feel "locked in" with their patients, for their relationships with one another can go on for decades and are not limited by a six- or eight-session maximum. Because of this, and linked to it, primary care physicians often have to worry about pleasing their patients. They have an incentive to prescribe medicines when patients want them, to order tests when patients request them, to see the patients even if their schedule is very tight, to take blood pressures on request, and so on— or else the patient will go elsewhere. Of course, the physician may try to educate the patient to his or her own perspective. But, failing the success of this at any given moment, physicians usually have to deal with reality as their patients present it, not as they would like it to be presented. This leads to a deeply ambivalent relationship between patient and physician, a relationship that has only been intensified, in recent years, by the willingness of the patient (or the patient's family) to become a plaintiff if the outcome of medical care is not what they want. Because they know this, and because physicians are legally responsible for treatment, even that rendered by their secretaries and assistants, many physicians wind up being wary, frightened and close-mouthed around their patients with problems. Social workers are usually in no such comparable legal jeopardy. Indeed, whereas physician tend to keep much information to themselves, social workers' occupational values reward sharing of information and building an "honest" and open relationship.

Physicians in private practice are financially dependent on their patients for their livelihood. This often makes them more likely to grant what their patients ask of them. The same is not true of social workers. They may see their job as helping their clients get what the system owes them, but they are not dependent on their clients for their jobs, but rather to the agencies that employ them. The same may not be true for social workers, it must be pointed out, who are counselors and therapists in a private practice setting.

Therapists, like physicians, are dependent on their patients for their income. But they possess skills that can help them distance themselves from the relationship with their patients. They can talk about transference phenomena, can view any unpleasant traits the patient exhibits as "part of the problem." Most physicians do not do this. They tend to react more subjectively to the patients' behavior, and to see their patients as good patients and bad patients much more than do therapists.

The general practitioner occupies a position midway between the lay and the specialist referral systems. The social worker is not in a comparable position. This often leads the physician to feeling on the line between family, patient and specialists, between family and hospital, and so on. The social worker's allegiance seems clearer, and the limitations on his or her work also seem easier to define.

Finally, the disciplines have different views about the practice of collaborative care itself.

Huntington points out that medicine and social work view one another differently. Physicians tend to view social workers (and other helpers) as auxiliary wheels. Social workers, like other members of the health care team, often idealize physicians and—even though they get into furious disputes with them—accept their leadership position. Changes in the composition of social work, such as more men entering the field, and the shifts in consciousness wrought by the women's movement, may well alter the relationship between the two fields in collaboration. Central to this is the social workers' understanding the nature of the physicians' work:

> If social workers were more aware of the forces shaping the nature of the general practitioner-patient relationship, the behavior and attitudes of general practitioners would be more intelligible. Perhaps it is more comfortable for social work not to try to understand these forces, because to do so would bring social work face to face with powerful, unresolved aspects of its own identity and practice (Huntington, 1981, p. 124).

In trying to help physicians and social workers collaborate more effectively, Huntington suggests that there are different types of general practitioner physicians, marked by differences in their overall orientation—for example, GP as father figure, GP as family doctor, GP as psychophysician, and so on—as well as different types of social workers—paramedic, psychotherapist, agent of change at the micro level. She further suggests that certain types of physicians will find it more easy to collaborate with social workers—and particularly with some types of social workers—than will others. This kind of analysis appears potentially fruitful. It brings to mind some of the work done on "world outlook" by Bibace (personal communication), which shows that physicians will tend to have patients whose general world view mirrors their own. If this is true for the working compatibility of physicians and patients, it is probably equally true for the compatibility of physicians and potential colleagues in health care—social workers, therapists, and so on.

MEDICAL CARE VERSUS "SOCIAL CARE"

Moving from this general discussion, we can start applying Huntington's ideas to the settings with which we are personally familiar. To start with, both social work and general medicine have had a tendency to define themselves more broadly in recent years. The impact of the biopsychosocial model of illness has made it possible for medicine to claim responsibility for many psychosocial problems, the consequences of which extend into the area of health and illness. Social workers, long used to bearing the responsibility for "social problems," have increasingly entered the health care arena. This has led to some over-lap in what each field feels is appropriate to its own concern. Without a clear-cut definition of role, then, in any given practice, there will be room for dispute over turf and territory.

My feeling is that Huntington's analysis has laid the foundation for the next stage in collaborative health care, a stage marked by people's moving cautiously ahead to explore how they can work together in both public and private sectors. Job descriptions must be clear. Issues have to be on the table for open discussion. Differences have to be acknowledged, but at the same time a common purpose, a common vision needs also to be accepted. This is a stage that is already being entered, I think, by social worker writers such as Gregory Greene, whose several papers deal with new opportunities for social workers in family practice and who has suggested the new term "family practice social worker" (Greene et al., 1985).

But there are other, broader questions. Which, really, is the principal service—medical or social care? Whose role is it to provide such care—the government or the entrepreneurial class? When a program is organized, who is its leader—the executive director, the physician, or the staff person with the best systemic perspective? What is the relationship between health care sites and the communities they serve? Are health care sites entrepreneurial businesses that offer health care for sale, or are they seen more as a part of their community, working in some form of partnership with the people who live there? Such dichotomies stem from different concepts of social organization and involve conflicting hierarchies of wants and values. These issues, essentially "extrinsic" to health team practice, are critical, for they set the rules for whatever kinds of practices can exist.

SUMMARY

The present time offers an opportunity for the reorganization of health care services. Economic, social, and political pressures have all come to focus on medical care, and some drastic changes are clearly called for. Collaborative health care offers a model of comprehensive care that is at the same time cost-effective, integrated, community-based, and pleasing to patients. Even so, many factors act to prevent CHC from making greater inroads: (1) Some people remember the collaborative experience of the 1960s as a failure; (2) The advocates of specialty, fragmented medical care are strong; (3) The biomedical model has gained new strength, buttressed by the DRGs, the diagnostic codes now in use, the fee structures and their reimbursement regulations of all third-party insurance programs (from Blue Shield-Blue Cross to Medicaid and Medicare); (4) Where attempts at collaborative care have been tried, a number of intrinsic conflicts over money, power, and overall perspective have risen, and it is difficult to keep such care going without support at a higher governmental level. People tend to burn out if acting on their values means going against their own self-interest, without support, day after day.

It would appear that broader support from government officials and policymakers will only emerge when the advocates of collaborative care can show two things: (1) that collaborative practices can indeed deal with their internal difficulties, and, more importantly, (2) that such care is in the public interest. That is, we need to have data from some current sentinal practices showing that comprehensive care does in fact promote people's health, prevent illness, and save money in the long run. Once this information is available, printed, and popularized, it will have a chance of greater acceptance.

ELEVEN

Referral to the Therapist

Many practical problems arise in collaborative health care. One of the most basic ones concerns referral. How will the physician and the counselor move patients from one to the other and back, and coordinate their care. Many practitioners just starting out are concerned about getting off on the right foot, and the referral process seems a suitable place to begin answering their questions. When is a referral called for? How is a referral best made?

THE REFERRAL PROCESS IN GENERAL

Referrals take place all the time in medical practice. Generalists refer to specialists; specialists refer to one another. Medical sociologists have divided medical practice into client-dependent (as for family physicians) and colleague-dependent (as for most specialists) (Freidson, 1970); these concepts help clarify some of the issues involved in the etiquette of the referral process.

Family physicians want the best for their patients. They refer a patient to a specialist when they feel a problem at hand demands specialist expertise, when a very difficult decision needs to be made, or when treatment issues are exceedingly complex. A good family physician is not afraid to refer when necessary.

Generalists, of course, do not want to refer everybody. They enjoy diagnosis and treatment and they pride themselves on being able to handle most of their patients' problems. In addition, they know that some young specialists will "steal" patients. Some specialists denigrate the family physician. Some try to take patients away, through their access to emergency rooms, cardiac care units, and such, from which the family physician may be excluded, and so on. There is thus a material basis for the family physician's reluctance to refer unnecessarily. Primary care physicians have become distrustful of specialists as a group, though less so of the few trusted specialist colleagues to whom most of their referrals flow.

Patients differ in what they expect of their physician. Some insist on specialist care for any complaint they consider serious; others will want second opinions before surgery; others will want a specialist for their children, but not for themselves; or for some organ system problems but not for others. This is an individual matter that physicians must respect, so far as the organization of their practice permits.

Physician differ, too, in their abilities and interests. Some family physicians prefer to keep active in surgical work; others in ob-gyn; others in family counseling. Referrals, in other words, will vary from physician to physician. The main determinants of a rational approach to referral are: (1) not referring any patient unnecessarily, and (2) not holding back from any referral when indicated.

THE THERAPY REFERRAL

Referrals to counselors and therapists are often fraught with tension. One source is a lack of contact and a shared approach on the part of the two professionals. Physicians and therapists frequently talk two different languages, and there are other differences between the professions. The best referrals happen when generalist and specialist see problems in a similar way. Family physicians with a family perspective will usually want to refer to a family-oriented therapist; family physicians with a more traditional approach will refer to more traditionally oriented psychiatrists or psychologists.

If the therapy specialist is not affiliated with the medical practice, a therapy referral immediately confronts several difficulties:

- The patient may perceive the referral as a rejection;
- The patient may perceive the referral as a statement that s/he is crazy;
- The patient's family may come into conflict with both the referral and the therapist;
- The therapist may be working at odds with the family doctor, may not share the same approach, may not communicate to the family doctor. When the therapist is more traditional, and the family physician

is more inclined toward a family perspective, the therapist may actually work at cross purposes with the physician. This may result in an unhelpful triangulation, as described by Doherty and Baird (1983). It may also lead to the same kind of unintentional scapegoating the discovery of which family therapy arose so much against;

• Compliance with a referral for therapy "across town" is abysmally low. Between 50 and 90 percent of those referred will not keep the appointment.

Having a therapist within the practice deals with many of these problems. Certainly, compliance is much higher within a collaborative practice—in our practice, close to 90 percent. Communication is much easier to accomplish. And, hopefully, a shared orientation exists between therapists and physicians. And yet, there are still problems around the therapy referral, and what it signifies to the patient, the physician, and the therapist.

TACIT PROBLEMS REGARDING THE REFERRAL

Even in a well-run collaborative practice, patients may experience the therapy referral—especially when it is accompanied by obvious frustration on the physician's part—as a rejection and dismissal. Physicians need to learn how to reframe their frustration when they refer, to speak of their sense of helplessness while acknowledging their desire to help the patient. They should also outline plans for maintaining contact and continuing to provide care. This will help the patient from feeling cast aside. Often, a simple acknowledgement that, "I'm starting to feel that there's more involved in this than I can cope with," may be a good place to start. So might the statement that, "I feel that I'm not being as helpful to you now as I'd like to be, and I think that's because of _____." Whatever words the physician cares to use, the message can be given that more is needed than he or she can provide, and that's why they want a consultation.

Physicians' attitudes toward emotional problems in general frequently surface around their referrals. Do physicians think people ought to handle their own problems? If so, do they feel a sense of failure when they have to make a referral to the therapist, having failed to solve the problem by themselves. Do they communicate this to the patient? Are patients really given up on when referred to the therapist, or are they still eagerly followed, in the genuine desire to learn something further about the problems and how to treat them. Patients quickly intuit their physicians' biases.

Similarly, patients pick up the therapists' opinions about whether emotional problems affect one's general worth.

One pitfall regarding referral can be called "the trap of premature closure." If the physician feels the problem is already defined, and/or if the patient and the patient's family feel the problem is already defined, then they may unwittingly present a resistance to the therapist's need to widen the horizons, question all assumptions, and make a new start at defining the problem and its solution.

THE PHYSICIAN'S MANA

The physician possesses a magical power, which can sometimes be transferred to the therapist. In a family practice, collaborating professionals may be experienced by the patients as the physician's brothers or sisters. When the physician tells the patient, "Go and see _____. She is an excellent counselor, and I think she'll be able to help you," a transference of mana occurs, a transfer of the physician's aura and power. This is even more powerful when the physician physically brings patients to meet the therapist, thus literally "handing them over." The transfer-of-hands carries a powerful religious and healing significance.

The existence of perceived family-like relationships among the staff in a family medical practice acts to reinforce and support all referrals within that practice. It also sets the stage for unhelpful triangulation—just like in families—if therapist and physician do not communicate.

WHEN TO REFER

Candib has pointed out (1985) that previous criteria for identifying "difficult patients" in family practice now appear equally well to represent criteria for convening the family as well as criteria for making a referral for family therapy.

Schmidt's Criteria for Convening the Family

Schmidt (1983) has listed a number of conditions for when convening the family might be useful. These include: pregnancy, failure to thrive, recurrent childhood poisoning, school and preschool behavior problems, adolescent maladjustment, major depression, chronic illness, diabetes, coronary bypass surgery, myocardial infarction, poor adherence to the medical regimen, high "inapproprate" use of health services, terminal illness, and bereavement.

Ransom and Grace's Conditions for Which
Family Treatment Is Indicated

Ransom and Grace (1979) list a dozen conditions for which family treatment is indicated. These include: marital and sexual adjustment problems which are presented as such in the office; family problems brought up as needing attention; any problem involving children that is greater than a self-limiting or common illness; serious problems of teenagers; a crisis or chaos in the family that is not being well-handled and that may lead to further distress or symptomatic behavior; when one person in the family claims that the problem is caused by another; when any member of the family shows signs of mental or emotional disturbance; when any member develops a stress-related illness; when intervention requires life-style changes affecting or involving other members of the family; when a serious, chronic illness or disability in a member is not being handled well by the family; when medical symptoms are present for which no organic basis can be found; and when other forms of treatment have failed.

Candib's Insight

Candib, looking at the lists of conditions for which a family approach is suggested, observed that these were the very same conditions which the founders of family medicine (compare Stephens, 1982) claimed required a therapeutic relationship with the family physician. "Thus," she observes (1984), "the kinds of problems of individuals which originally defined the content of family practice are being redefined as problems of families."

It would appear that "when to refer" and "what problems to refer" are both questions in the process of being renegotiated. Different family physicians will choose different conditions for referral and different times for such referral. There does however seem to be some overall agreement that a consideration of family-oriented treatment and/or a referral for therapy should occur whenever:

- The patient's symptoms seem unexplained by medical findings;
- The problem appears to involve other members of the family;
- Noncompliance of any kind is developing;
- The physician feels over his head with some emotional or relational problem presented by the patient;
- The physician feels helplessly triangulated between family members;

- The physician feels helplessly in conflict with the patient over diagnostic or treatment issues;
- The patient's problem appears to significantly coincide with a stage in the family's developmental cycle;
- The patient's problem involves discovery of cancer, sudden change in physical health, or death;
- A cloak of secrecy, of great significance and weight, seems cast over some critical family member;
- Obvious emotional difficulties are presented by the patient in the course of treatment.

As more and more practices involve therapists working side by side with physicians, one might expect even more problems to be deemed appropriate for evaluation by the therapist. After all, every human existence involves change and stress, and the therapist is presumably adept at helping people deal with such stress; and so the therapist's evaluation of individual and/or the family may always be appropriate, given the availability of such resources. More importantly, such collaborative practices will have to show that a good deal of time and money can be saved by evaluating families periodically and intervening prospectively. Currently, however, studies that document this savings are scanty and more needs to be done.

For now, let us say that the indications for referral have generally been set forth. What remains is for collaborative teams to act on these indications; to intervene; and to report the results of such intervention.

It should also be pointed out that some family physicians will be more inclined than others to treat patients with psychosocial or psychosomatic difficulties. They may thus refer a smaller percentage of patients with such difficulties to the therapist, choosing instead to treat more of the patients on their own. At the same time, if our own practice is any indication of tendencies among physicians, simply noting the existence of psychosocial and psychosomatic problems leads the physician to "discover" more such problems among the patients in his or her practice, and may thus lead to increased overall use of the collaborating therapist. This is certainly the case in our own practice, for even though the physicians treat at least half of all patients with psychosocial difficulties themselves, our referrals to the therapist went up so sharply that a second therapist had to be found, and then that therapist had to arrange for an assistant; and still we had greater need for counseling services than we could ourselves provide.

This whole question of when and what will be further refined over the coming ten years.

Huygen's Insights

Huygen, who works with family therapists in the department of general practice of the Nijmegen University, in the Netherlands, has discussed the general topic of family therapy in family practice in his *Family Medicine* (1978). Having become convinced that family therapy was a necessary collaborative adjunct to family medical practice, his department started a systematic collaboration with the Department of Family Therapy. At the time he wrote his monograph, 300 families had been treated collaboratively in this way.

Huygen makes a distinction very early between family therapy and other available forms of psychotherapy. The effects of the "usual kind of psychotherapy" are "disappointing" (p. 134). Family therapy, by addressing the broader social context in which the patient lives, "offers a possibility to break and modify this chain of events [that is, generational patterns] as it is not primarily directed at individuals but at their mutual relationships" (p. 134). It also "opens up the perspective of prevention" (p. 134).

Huygen presents two case histories to illustrate the ways the therapists can highlight family processes for the family physician. In the first, the therapist refused to be cowed by the patient's persistent somatic complaints, through which she had for years dominated and controled both her family and her family physician: "The family therapists thwarted her in turn by stating in the very first interview that they realized that she was in such a bad state that they did not think they would be able to help her. The only thing they could try to do was help Mrs. Poppy and her family to live with her symptoms."

Mrs. Poppy did not like this and "revolted" against the therapists. Her symptoms worsened. She became gravely depressed. The therapists did not relent, but they showed consistent concern for Mrs. Poppy's distress, even to the point of, when she threatened suicide, talking "at length with her over the way she was going to do this, how and where, what kind of dress she would be wearing and so on. They asked her about the kind of burial ceremony she wanted and what she thought about the impact on her family. Mrs. Poppy went through hell but to my astonishment and great relief shortly afterwards came out of it as though reborn" (p. 136).

Huygen refers to family therapy as having proved to be a "kind of adventure" for the GPs. "The family therapists challenged and rated our patients higher than we were used to doing as their general practitioners" (p. 137).

Huygen then summarizes what he learned from his collaboration with family therapists. The following points come out in his discussion (the numbering is my own):

1. It is easier to refer individuals than families. Let the therapist take care of involving the families and motivating them for therapy.

2. To motivate patients for family therapy, "it was better to start from the worries about symptoms and the consequences of disturbances . . . for the other family members, than to start from a search for causes of these disturbances in the family" (p. 138). A search for "causes" creates resistance.

3. Family therapists worked with "here and now" phenomena and tried to involve everyone in the family. They "worked with very limited numbers of sessions, after which they referred the patients back to the GP with instructions on how to proceed" (p. 138). It was usually left open that, if further problems arose, the patient could see the therapist again. But brief treatment appeared to encourage the patient and family's self-reliance.

4. "The best moment to refer to family therapy proved to be times of crisis." Capacity for change seems greatest at crisis points. To this end, family therapists "often intentionally provoke crises, *making cooperation between therapist and family doctor indispensable to prevent conflicting lines of conduct in the treatment of these families.* [italics mine]"

5. "Often it will be necessary to agree in dividing the different roles in the strategy of approach between family therapist and family doctor."

Cooperation with family therapists taught the physicians to look at families more intensively. It also resulted in some surprise improvements for families until then felt to have little chance of such change.

Huygen made an attempt to measure the results of therapy intervention objectively. He measured number of referrals to specialists, number of visits to the family physician, and number of prescriptions written. He concluded that family therapy intervention helped make the treated families more self-reliant. The number of contacts with the GP diminished significantly not only for the identified patient but also for the rest of the family members. The same held for the number of prescriptions for psychoactive drugs. Both the treating physicians and the patients themselves reported improvement in the patients' overall health. This was so even though the actual number of family therapy sessions had been quite small—four or five on average.

Christie-Seely's Contribution

Christie-Seely (1984) describes the family physician's "working with the family." "Rarely," she comments, "a family will need or request more intensive intervention"; and she goes on to discuss referrals for family therapy. My sense is that collaborative care can involve the family counselor with much more of the routine counseling work, and that the family therapy referral need not be so rare. In our own practice, about half to two-thirds of what might be called situational problems are still handled by the primary care physician, and perhaps an even higher percentage of seriously disturbed patients. Even so, a high percentage of difficult situational problems, as well as many characterological and even neurotic disorders are referred to the family therapist. More yet are referred when physicians become very busy.

Christie-Seely's discussion of referral starts off with the most difficult of all patients to refer, the "psychosomatic family" (p. 252). "A psychosomatic family, because of its rigidity and avoidance of conflicts, is both very difficult to treat and to refer," she notes. (Our experience would have us add that these families use projection and denial a great deal—combined, these foster somaticization—and are thus difficult to "hook.")

She then notes the importance of the physician's maintaining contact with the therapist, so that neither undermines the work of the other. This is true, but her discussion does not address the question of collaborative care in one's practice; rather, she seems to assume that the physician is referring his or her patients out.

Christie-Seely gives several indications for a therapy referral, beginning with the list given by Bullock and Thompson (1979): (1) history of repeated attempts at therapy; (2) missed appointments; (3) commitment to sessions as a family unit but at no session does everyone attend; (4) long duration of dysfunction pattern; (5) refusal to pay prescribed fees; (6) no improvement after five or six sessions. To this, she adds: (7) serious problems in more than one family member; (8) more than one serious problem in a child with behavioral difficulties; (9) changing doctors often and refusing to agree to drop all other physicians or health care contacts; and (10) when a patient has developed too strong an alliance with the patient or one family member and cannot be objective in assessment and intervention.

She underscores the role of the family physician's continuing with the patient and family during and after the referral, so that they have no sense of being abandoned. (This is naturally done in a collaborative setting, where the physician obviously continues to see the patient and family.)

Advice from Doherty and Baird

A referral for counseling is appropriate when there is evidence of disturbed family functioning. Doherty and Baird (1983) list several "common clinical presentations" that suggest such disturbed family functioning. These include: (1) "Atypical migraine" headaches of long-standing duration; (2) persons with chronic depression, unmanageable by any long-term therapy, either medical or electroconvulsive; (3) the patient presenting with "chronic anxiety" who has had many office visits over several years for multiple and diffuse complaints without significant diagnostic evidence of "organic" disease; (4) patients presenting with a primary complaint of chronic fatigue; (5) a number of pediatric complaints for which educating the parents has not been effective ("poor appetite" in the first year of life, despite a healthy appearance; reported poor sleep patterns in one-year-olds; reported "hyperactivity" but the child behaves well in the office); insomnia in certain patients. Generally speaking, they conclude, "any consistent complaint that defies medical explanation after repeated examinations . . . may be a clue to family dysfunction" (p. 48). Doherty and Baird do not feel all these patients should necessarily be referred for therapy. Indeed, they feel primary care physicians should be doing a good deal of counseling themselves, what Doherty and Baird call "primary care counselling." Failing this, a referral for therapy might well be indicated.

Looking at our own practice, I would agree with psychosocial attention for these categories. In fact, family dysfunction and psychological difficulties may be intuited even before extensive medical workup. Patients, of course, may think that physical complaints only go with physical illness. Often, however, the physician must pursue a comprehensive medical workup in order to convince the patient that a recommended referral for therapy is warranted. This may be true when the physicians carry out such counseling themselves, as well as when they refer the patient to a therapist.

The subject of referral merits a whole chapter in Doherty and Baird's book. They begin with a discussion of the referral process in general, then note that dangers can arise from referring too late as well as from too early. In the first instance, the family physician may end up ineffectively treating psychosocial problems that should have been referred to a counselor. In the second, the family physician "fail[s] to offer immediate help to patients and families by making inappropriate or premature referrals to the specialized mental health sector" (p. 76).

Doherty and Baird's antidote to this is a rule of thumb: The family physician will refer a patient or family to a therapist "if the problem is not ameliorated through primary care counseling." The general intent of the rule is clear: Physicians should handle many psychosocial problems themselves, but should not get badly over their heads. In practice, this "rule" turns out to be no rule at all. Physicians who enjoy treating psychosocial problems themselves will do so unless they have no time or until they feel that a problem is beyond them. Physicians who have not learned counseling skills will be satisfied to recognize that a problem exists for which they will appropriately refer the patient and family.

Doherty and Baird sometimes fail to acknowledge the complexity of things. Thus, for example, they imply that therapy is a specialized form of interaction, appropriate only to difficult problems, whereas primary care counseling is more easily learned, less deep, and part of the physicians' repertoire. This avoids seeing that therapists and counselors possess a great number of skills, some of which are useful in intervening in very brief and delimited situations, others of which may be useful for longer period of interaction. Not all therapy, not even all family therapy is alike. Dividing therapy into the simpler skills (primary care counseling) and the more difficult skills (therapy) overlooks the fact that brief counseling may be a difficult skill, that therapy itself may be framed as open-ended, goal-oriented, brief-term, ten sessions long (because of insurance or other regulations), and so on. They beg the question, At what level is a trained therapist's skill most helpful to the patient? At what point does it surpass whatever the physician can offer?

They would, however, correctly have physicians first assess the situation in which psychosocial problems arise, then try dealing with the psychosocial problems themselves—as time and training permit—("primary care counseling"). Then, if the problem does not seem improved, or if its solution seems to demand a greater level of skill than they possess, they will refer to the therapy specialist.

This notion of levels has been elaborated by Doherty elsewhere (1985).

They note that, when physicians make a referral, they should attempt to reach agreement with the patient about it first, and should also meet with the family. They point out that a referral has a better chance of success if the family has come together around it. "Referring a family is best accomplished at a family meeting" (p. 77).

On further reflection, it isn't obvious that a family meeting is always advisable. I can think of several scenarios where the physician's main task is to get the patient to a therapist and let the therapist decide whom to involve. For example, a wife who is depressed over her marriage may not get into therapy at all if the physician first tries to bring the husband to a meeting before he is ready. It may be better to let the therapist recruit the other members of the family. Much of this depends on the physician's relationships with others in the family, on the nature of the "family practice" being discussed, on the patient's wishes, and on the skill of the physician at joining people in a common effort and at organizing people into a common venture.

Some patients may not want their family to be involved in treatment from the very beginning, even if this is ultimately the necessary step they must take. For this reason, I would question always assembling the family in order to make a therapy referral. My guideline would be, ask family members to come when it seems right, and use the facts of who comes as a communication about the family to be relayed on to the therapist.

Doherty and Baird next give criteria for deciding to treat or to refer. These criteria are:

1. The nature of the problem. Generally speaking, serious, chronic psychosocial problems should be referred. These include: chronic depression and anxiety that have not responded to previous biomedical or psychotherapeutic treatment; chemical dependency; chronic family dysfunctional patterns, and serious acute family symptoms such as child abuse, spouse abuse, and incest. On the other hand, some kinds of problems are generally appropriate for primary care counseling by a primary care physician, including family transition problems; other problems of recent origin; and many illness-related problems. Of course, they point out, many problems that seem simple and mild are

actually complex and severe, and one realizes that as one begins to work.

2. The physician's knowledge and ability—his or her level of training and command of skills, as well as interest in doing this kind of counseling work.

3. The physician's time and resources to take on such counseling.

The two also consider the art of referring. Central to their discussion is the notion of a "referral triangle." This is a three-sided relationship similar to the physician-patient-family therapeutic triangle. It includes the physician, the patient (and patient's family), and the consultant. If the physician has not engaged the family in a single-minded way, of course, the triangle opens up into some multi-sided figure, with the increasing likelihood of those numerous conflicting triangular relationships with which we are all familiar: mother/patient/consultant versus father/brother/physician; patient/physician/consultant versus sister/father/grandma; patient/grandma/physician versus mother/father/consultant; and so on.

When the triangle is "simple," Doherty and Baird point out, other relationships may not have a chance to develop. For example, the patient/physician relationship may be too intense, too "enmeshed" to permit the consultant access to the patient. A "disengaged" patient/physician relationship, in which the physician has not done the work of establishing rapport with the patient and/or family, is "unlikely to give birth to a triad" (p. 82), that is, is unlikely to bring the patient into another relationship with the therapist consultant.

Similarly, the physician and therapist need to know and trust one another. Otherwise each might undermine the other's treatment, or a manipulative patient might skillfully exploit their differences. But how does the physician learn to trust the therapist/consultant? Doherty and Baird suggest that primary care and family physicians should refer to therapists with a family orientation. That is, physicians with a biopsychosocial perspective should refer to therapists who share such a systemic world view; and these therapists are likely to be family therapists at this point in time.

The guidelines Doherty and Baird draw out cannot be taken as fixed, but are in fact rules of thumb, suggestions. The main determinants of the referral process are the physician's own interests, skills and training, the amount of time available, and the type of outside resources available for the referral. Given this caveat, their criteria are helpful.

There is no substitute, of course, for physicians' making decisions based on their own interaction with the problem. One must interact with the patient and the problem, try to produce some change, some insight, some clarity by observing, questioning, interacting, confronting, and so on. How long one has to do this before deciding that a problem requires referral is a matter that will vary from physician to physician, depending on level of training, age, time available, life goals, level of psychosocial sensitivity, and so on.

PRACTICAL TIPS

Some simple aspects of the referring process can increase the chance of success. Where possible, the referring physician should help structure the patient's contact with the therapist. If the patient is shy, the physician might bring him or her over to the therapist and introduce them. If the patient is ambivalent, the physician might acknowledge that a decision to accept a referral for therapy is an initial (positive) step in the therapeutic process (which it is, anyway). If the patient has had a previous "bad" experience with a therapist—"He kept looking at me and never talked!" "I went for two months, and nothing changed!"—the physician could ask about what made it so unpleasant, and could say concretely how the current therapist quite likely differs from the previous one.

Another potentially important factor is gender. The referring physician should sense whether the patient would do better with a male or female therapist. If the practice is small, for instance, with only a male therapist working alongside the physician, and if the physician feels that the patient needs a female therapist, it may be advisable to refer that patient to an outside therapist, rather than insist on her seeing the therapist in the practice. Similarly, the age of the therapist may be an important consideration. A physician should sense which therapists are available, either within the practice or outside it, to treat the range of needs that might arise. In our own practice, we were once fortunate in having two women therapists—one in her thirties, one in her forties—and two men—one in his late twenties and one in his thirties. That gave us more options than we might otherwise have had.

Of course, many times the therapist's age or sex is not a main concern. Usually the principal difficulties faced by the referring physician stem from the patient's worries about therapy. Whatever the physician can honestly do or say to diminish these worries and bring the patient to the therapist's office will be a step forward.

Once the patient has reached the therapist, it is up to the latter to "join" with the patient and assess the problem at hand, offering the patient treatment if it is felt appropriate. The skills useful to this endeavor have been well covered in the therapy literature.

TWELVE

Questions Frequently Asked about CHC

This chapter attempts to answer some of the more common questions readers have about collaborative health care.

1. *What kind of charts and records do you keep in a collaborative practice?*

The most helpful, the most informative records integrate all modes of treatment. We use a family chart which contains all the individual medical records of the people in a single family or household. The chart may contain a sheet with a "family problem list" as well. Individual charts contain individual problem lists. Our staff is supposed to send a patient's entire family chart in to the practitioner each time that patient is seen.

We think therapists should write notes in the combined health record. This can be in an individual patient's chart or it may be on a separate sheet attached to the family folder. The notes don't have to be long (in fact, it's better if they're not). It's usually enough to write notes one or two paragraphs long, summing up what happened at the last session, putting forth a plan or change of plan, or sharing critical information. In our practice, the therapist writes on the same yellow continuation sheets as the physicians use, thus creating a chronological record of all health encounters. In other practices, therapists may write in a separate section of the chart. The chart can be organized in whatever way makes sense for the practice. If you are going to use the charts for research purposes—that is, to answer questions such as, "Do physician visits drop after a referral to the counselor?"—you should organize your charts so that you can retrieve this kind of information.

Therapists often keep two sets of notes. One set goes into the chart; it briefly summarizes the treatment work and treatment plan, sets forth salient issues, and alerts other members of the practice to any possible problems. The other set of notes may be more detailed. It is actually the therapist's personal notes and observations of the session, as well as his or her private thoughts; such material is best kept privately in the therapist's office.

The practice may also keep billing information separately on the patient and/or family on a simple ledger card or computer file.

2. *How do you handle questions of confidentiality?*

This is a very complex question. Some practices get a written consent form from the patient, giving the counselor and the physician permission to discuss treatment issues conjointly. We don't have such a form, but it's understood that physicians and counselors will be discussing the patient together from time to time. Material that might embarrass the patient—matters relating to sexual fantasies, childhood traumatic events—or that has no relevant purpose for being written in the chart—lengthy descriptions of past events, dream material—is kept out of it; if such material seems pertinent to medical treatment, it can be communicated verbally.

We try to write as little as possible in the charts, but at the same time try to put all the information there that we need for medical and legal purposes. We recognize that our charts may be summoned by lawyers, insurance companies, and others, so we try to keep "personal" material out of them. We feel data such as the physician's own reaction to the patient is often appropriate, and I will sometimes include it in my notes under the section which contains "objective" data. (Using the S-O-A-P form, one writes the patient's *S*ubjective complaints and statements, describes the *O*bjective, observed findings, records an *A*ssessment of the problem, and then formulates a *P*lan.) I sometimes draw a diagram showing family patterns of interaction that I've observed in the encounter, or I may comment on the feelings the patient elicits from me in the "O" section. Our therapists frequently find this helpful.

Statements regarding suspicion of substance abuse or illicit activity must, of course, if written at all, be written specifically as a matter of personal speculation. Hearsay information about patients may at times be relevant ("wife says patient is not taking his medicines"), but it must be labeled for what it is.

We feel obliged to hear information about our patients from anyone who calls up and wishes to speak to us about them. But we also feel obliged to share this information with our patients. We are under no obligation to tell a relative or friend of a patient *anything* about their medical or emotional status, without the patient's permission. Exceptions may of course be made—to the most immediate members of an ill patient's family, or when a life-or-death question is at hand. *Example.* On her routine medical visit, Mrs. R. said she was worried about her son Kevin, and asked if the therapist treating him had spoken to me about him. I asked why. She said, because Kevin had been going around the house moodily lately, talking about "blowing his brains out," and this kind of suicidal talk was upsetting her. I put the information in the chart and flagged the chart for the therapist. The next day the therapist told me that he'd spoken to Kevin about it, and the boy had not seemed suicidal at all to him. He felt it was an example of the mother's trying to "triangle" the physician in the on-going family dispute over "who was to blame for the main problem," in other words, who's really the "sick" one. He planned to involve the mother more strongly in the next treatment sessions.

3. *What happens if a patient tries to set the physician against the therapist and vice versa?*

This happens often, especially with borderline patients who excel in "splitting." The only way of dealing with it is for both therapist and physician to recognize when it is happening. Sometimes, with a patient who uses medical/physical symptoms to avoid dealing with emotional issues, it may be wise to defuse possible conflict by defining the situation as mainly a counselling issue and failing to become frantic over endless somatic complaints. If problems persist, a session together may help clarify what's really going on.

4. *How often should the therapist and physician meet? Should this be regular?*

This depends on the kind of practice you have, and on how closely you want to work together. We find it useful to have a regular time each week for therapists and physicians to get together. The agenda for this meeting can vary from a case discussion, to reading an article and discussing it together, to simply talking about how things are going in the office. Therapists and physicians have many items to discuss—

treatment issues, their own process, problems with the support staff, as well as administrative issues, future plans, projects, anecdotes, and dealing with mutual tensions. In some practices, ours for instance, the therapists and physicians like to spend some social time together with their spouses, too. Other practices may prefer a strictly business relationship. In any case, we find that a regular meeting time is an important part of the week, and if it is part of everyone's schedule, it will be used for sharing information.

Many meetings also take place informally, if people are in the office together. People will catch one another in the halls, by the coffee machine, in one another's offices. Being available is one of the most important traits for people working in a successful collaborative arrangement.

5. *How do you deal with urgent issues, if they involve both a physician and a therapist?*

First, we try always to write relevant material in the chart and, if necessary, flag it for the other person. We may leave a chart on someone else's desk, or we may leave a note on that person's bulletin board or "IN" box. Second, we leave notes for one another during the day, giving important information and asking the other to stop by for a brief chat before the day is over. Third, we trap one another in the hall or kitchen during break or lunch times. Fourth, if necessary, we phone one another and discuss the problem. If an urgent decision has to be made and the other isn't available for some reason, we make the decision ourselves and notify the other one later.

6. *What happens when a patient has to be hospitalized for psychiatric reasons?*

The answer to this depends on the kind of practice you have and on the back-up resources available. If you are in an HMO that has psychiatric resources, then this is no problem; you follow your protocol. If you are in a small office, then you will need to speak to some psychiatrists in the area and prepare the way for their helping hospitalize any patients who need it, and serve as consultants when necessary for your patients. When it comes to psychiatric or substance-abuse hospitalization, patients (outside an HMO) usually split into two groups—those with insurance coverage and those without. Those without provide a real problem: Often you will have to go through the designated local mental health facility, whose staff may not share your own collaborative view of the problem. The best you can do is try to have open, collegial relationships with these other people and their institutions. Problems invariably arise, and people's tendency often is to blame someone else for a difficult situation. We try to avoid this and try to relate to other health professionals as if they had as much integrity as we like to think we do. Usually, this works out all right. Sometimes, though, a health professional from the local hospital or mental health clinic will make some disparaging remark about us or get involved with the patient or the family in a way that we feel works in the wrong direction. Sometimes there's nothing that can be done about it. Other times, we can try to talk.

I should add here that it's important to keep up a flow of information at all time; and therapists should know when their patients have been hospitalized for medical problems, too. Often, in fact, a medical hospitalization turns out to have a meaning in terms of the ongoing therapy, or has crucial consequences for other family members.

7. *What do you do if a medical patient can't afford therapy?*

Again, this kind of question only relates to people outside of HMOs. If people can't afford therapy, we try to see if there's a way they can work out something with the therapist over time. If there's no way a person, say, with Medicaid can see our therapist, then we have to refer that patient. We had asked Medicaid for years to include therapy in our office as part of covered services. Now, it seems, there's some chance that this might actually succeed; people are talking about enrolling all Medicaid recipients into HMOs in Massachusetts, and we would be part of one, with our capitation fee including therapy services. But, if the patient can't afford therapy care in a private setting, he or she has to be referred to the mental health clinics, unless the medical practice in some way is prepared to underwrite the cost of providing in-house therapy.

In passing, I should point out that the fragmentation of services has been institutionalized in our health care system. Most services are set up separately by specialty. Comprehensive care is hard to find in actual practice, and is often a battle to accomplish.

Physicians are fortunate enough to be reimbursable for most of their services, from almost all parties; and, in an HMO, they have a locked-in panel of patients whom they are paid to see. Therapists have to fight the discrimination of the closed-panel HMOs, the state (Medicaid) bureaucracy, and the licensing agencies. Frequently, since they cannot work for nothing, their ability to see patients is limited by the patient's income and/or insurance, as well as by the therapist's own capacity to negotiate fees and maneuver among the insurance diagnostic categories.

8. *Should every therapist have his or her own room?*

That depends on whether the therapist is working full-time in the practice. Usually, people like to have their own space. If a therapist is in a medical practice, it's better to have a room of one's own. Perhaps two part-time therapists might want to share the same room. Therapists who have their own office elsewhere, and who accept referrals from physicians, will of course have their own separate practices.

The issue of space is very meaningful, however. It will create relationships between the person who rents space and the one who owns it and will create the possibility for the therapist to have to pay a portion of his or her earnings for expenses (besides rent) such as the use of a common waiting room, phones and utilities, and office staff. If therapist and physician are on equal footing in this regard—that is, either both employees (of an HMO) or both partners (say, owning a collaborative health practice)—their relationship will be easier. Relationships resting on unequal power must be carefully defined; otherwise they will provide a source of mutual resentment and conflict.

9. *How do you handle conflict?*

There's bound to be conflict in any collaborative work. The best way to handle it is . . . to handle it! If you have a regular meeting time, you can discuss your conflicts then. It helps to have more than two people in the collaborative team, so no arguments wind up stuck one-on-one. It's always good to have another person free to come in and unstick things. It's also important to be able to deal with different kinds of conflicts. It's one thing to be able to talk about people's transference and counter-transference reactions and to speculate about family dynamics; it's another to be able to discuss social and political differences, different values systems, different sets of goals. I think conflict resolution begins with practitioners' feeling confident in their own ability, and also respecting their colleagues; conflict resolution depends on having an open mind and an acceptance of the differing voice.

10. *One potential area of conflict, for example: How do you handle the question of salary differences?*

The only way to handle this is to discuss it openly. Professionals assume different levels of responsibility for patient care, incur different costs (malpractice), and expect different incomes. Practices which encourage more equal sharing of their income will attract different personnel than those which accept different levels of income. The main criteria here is for people working together to have a shared understanding of this issue.

11. *What happens when the therapist and the physician disagree?*

People do disagree, and often. Therapists speak one language, physicians another; and people have different ways of looking at the world. Explanations about human experience and human interrelationships are often mutually compatible. In other words, our understanding of what makes people the way they are can usually be deepened by the ideas of people in fields other than our own, as well as by our own colleagues.

If there is disagreement over how to proceed, or what action to take, it has to be resolved one way or another. The best way of doing this is to discuss it openly and try to understand the different perceptions and opinions. If one person cannot be convinced, then the pair must agree on how to handle the disagreement. Is one person's word the "final" word? Do they seek out a third person to make a tie-breaking opinion? Do they take turns at yielding? This has to be built into the working arrangement. All in all, I think that disagreements over how to interpret some bit of behavior, or over the "real" diagnosis can usually be resolved by mutual discussion that clarifies the grounds (assumptions, perspective) for disagreement.

12. *How do you find funds to support collaborative practice?*

This is of course a central issue. If you are in private practice, you have to pay your way. Your therapy and counseling services are either reimbursable or they are not. If they are reimbursable, then these services pay their own way. But it often happens that the very services you most need to provide are not reimbursable. For example, the services of a nutritionist are rarely paid for by insurance companies, Medicare or Medicaid. The services of a social worker—who can help elderly or indigent patients with housing and transportation needs, assist them in navigating the welfare and disability bureaucracies, and find opportunities through job training and other educational programs—are not reimbursable. Physicians who want to include this in their practice may have to pay for it themselves, out of other sources of revenue.

At times, capitation programs for the poor and elderly may include enough additional revenue to pay the salaries of additional personnel, such as dieticians or social workers. These programs are few and far between, however, and physicians who participate in them may have to decide if additional services should be added to what the practice offers. In Great Britain, where physicians are under a capitation program, several GPs in a town may work together and pool their income, thus sharing the rent and overhead and having enough additional income to hire a social worker. The British program also provides financial incentives that encourage physicians in a group practice to hire ancillary health personnel, for example, underwriting a major part of these personnel's salaries, the remainder of which is a business expense. Such incentives are frequently lacking in the private sector in U.S. medicine, however.

The inequity of medical services in the United States is, of course, a serious impediment to comprehensive care. Whereas affluent patients can afford to pay for counseling and other associated services, those without money cannot. In our practice, most of the patients who need therapy services are on Medicaid, which will not pay our counselors (although it will pay an approved mental health center an exorbitant fee for counseling services). This kind of dilemma has no easy solutions.

Those practicing in clinic settings may be able to exert pressure in setting up the types of services offered. The same holds for those in HMOs. In the private sector, some of the more creative approaches have involved obtaining grants from foundations, accepting whatever payments patients can contribute to such extended care, and developing nonprofit foundations allied with the practice that then provide or purchase therapy and other ancillary services for the practice with money given as contributions.

THIRTEEN

Summary

Collaborative health care offers an interdisciplinary, systemic approach to health and disease. It rests on a working partnership between family-oriented physicians, counselors, and therapists, augmented as needed by other health professionals. This model of care can fit almost any setting—private or public, urban or rural, HMO or clinic. But it must be more widely known, and its practitioners need more material incentives and encouragement.

The concept has a rich past. It can draw upon many antecedents that give it credence and legitimacy. Its ideas are up to date, shaped by the latest theories and research. More than this, the recent confluence of professional interests—especially the rise of both family therapy and family medicine—has created the conditions in which collaborative care might actually flower. And yet, outside of teaching programs, collaborative care is still infrequently practiced. It still awaits its transformation from fancy into fact. The reasons behind this are mainly economic and cultural; they stem from intellectual timidity, the rise of businessmen's values in medicine, and the traditional in-fighting of entrenched professional cultures.

Here and there, of course, in private practices, clinics, HMOs, and training programs, physicians, therapists, social workers, and a variety of counselors and therapists have been nonetheless working together at providing a more comprehensive form of health care. Their efforts illuminate the process for others. Their successes can be copied; their shortcomings clarify the problems to be encountered.

Collaborative care is an excellent form of treatment for patients and their families, and it is also satisfying for the practitioner. It has the potential to monitor and contain costs more efficiently than any other form of health care organization so far, because CHC views health and illness in a broad and continuous—not narrow, episodic—context.

And yet old ways die hard. The medical world shows strong resistance to new forms of (especially, collaborative) organization. The focus today has shifted to forms of care that can bring in greater profits while containing third-party costs. Typically this has meant greater monopolization of health care services, an increasing corporatization of health care, sharper competition among providers, and steep cuts in covered services. Alternate ways of looking at the problem—focusing on preventive, more comprehensive services (the biopsychosocial approach)—have had little influence, and they lack funding and publicity. Existing financial incentives do not encourage their growth.

This book has presented an analysis of the ideas and experience that can shape collaborative health care today. It has examined earlier forms of collaborative care as well as some of the current practices where such care now exists. It has discussed a number of problems, both extrinsic and intrinsic to the collaborative process, and has suggested ways that CHC practitioners can grapple with these problems.

Collaborative health care can in fact become a reality if policymakers who see its promise can develop incentives and programs that encourage it. This struggle will take place over the next few years: will adherents of the broader view support their vision or abandon it? People who see health and illness in their natural/social context will need to participate in the dialogue between health care practitioners of all types and health policymakers or their view will not prevail.

BIBLIOGRAPHY

Abramson JH and Kark SL: "Community oriented primary care: Meaning and scope," in Connor E and Mullan F (Eds.): Community Oriented Primary Care: New Directions for Health Services Delivery. Washington, DC, National Academy Press, 1983, pp. 21-59.

Ader R: Psychoneuroimmunology. New York, Academic Press, 1981.

Antonovsky A: Health, Stress and Coping. San Francisco, Jossey-Bass, 1979.

Ashby WR: An Introduction to Cybernetics. London, Chapman and Hall, 1956.

Auerswald EH: The Gouverneur health services program: An experiment in ecosystemic community health care delivery. Family Systems Medicine *1*(2): 5-24, 1983.

Backett EM, Maybin RP, and Dudgeon Y: Medicosocial work in general practice. Lancet, *i*:37-40, 1957.

Balint M: The Doctor, His Patient and the Illness. New York, International Universities Press, 1957.

Banta HD and Fox RC. Role strains of a health care team in a poverty community. Social Science and Medicine *6*:697-722, 1972.

Bassoff BZ: "Collaboration in primary care: Or is it?" in Miller RS (Ed.): Primary Health Care: More Than Medicine. Englewood Cliffs (NJ), Prentice-Hall, 1983, pp. 123-132.

Bateson G, Jackson D, Haley J, and Weakland JH: Towards a theory of schizophrenia. Behavioral Science *1*:251-269, 1956.

Beavers WR: "Healthy, midrange, and severely dysfunctional families," in Walsh F (Ed.): Normal Family Processes. New York, Guilford Press, 1982, pp. 45-66.

Berkman L and Breslow L: Health and Ways of Living: The Alameda County Study. New York, Oxford University Press, 1983.

Bernard C: An Introduction to the Study of Experimental Medicine, translated by HC Greene. New York, Dover, 1957 (1927).

von Bertalanffy L: General System Theory. New York, Braziller, 1968.

Bhagat M, Lewis AP, and Shillitoe RW: The clinical psychologist and the primary health care team. Update *18*:479-484, 1979.

Bibace R: Personal communication, 1984.

Bishop DS: "Family therapy and family medicine," in Gurman AS (Ed.): Research and Clinical Exchange, American Journal of Family Therapy *9* (2): 89-91, 1981.

Black DB, Morrison J, Snyder LJ, and Tally P: Model for clinical social work practice in a health care facility. Social Work in Health Care *3*:143-148, 1977.

Bloch D: Personal communication, 1982.

Bloch D: Family systems medicine: The field and the journal. Family Systems Medicine *1*:3-11, 1983.

Borysenko M and Borysenko JZ: Stress, behavior and immunity. General Hospital Psychiatry *4*:59-67, 1982.

Bowen M: Family Therapy in Clinical Practice. New York, Jason Aronson, 1978.

Bracht NF: Social Work in Health Care: A Guide to Professional Practice. New York, Haworth, 1978.

Brochstein JR, Adams, GL, Tristan MP, and Chenbey CC: Social work and primary health care: An integrative approach. Social Work in Health Care *5*: 71-81, 1979.

Bruch H: Eating Disorders: Obesity, Anorexia, and the Person Within. New York, Basic Books, 1973.

Buckley W (Ed.): Modern Systems Research for the Behavioral Scientist. Chicago, Aldine, 1968.

Bullock D and Thompson B: Guidelines for family interviewing and brief therapy for the family physician. Journal of Family Practice *9*:837-841, 1979.

Candib LM: A Social Study of the Health Center Movement: A New Approach to Public Health History. Unpublished thesis, Harvard University, History of Science Department, 1968.

Candib LM: The family approach at each moment. Family Medicine *17*:201-208, 1985.

Candib LM and Glenn ML: Family medicine and family therapy: Comparative development, methods, and roles. Journal of Family Practice *16*:773-779, 1983.

Carmichael LP: Forty families: A search for the family in family medicine. Family Systems Medicine *1*(1):12-16, 1983.

Carmichael LP and Carmichael JS: The relational model in family practice. Marriage and Family Review *4*:123-134, 1981.

Christie-Seely J (Ed): Working with the Family in Primary Care. New York, Praeger, 1984.

Coleman JV, Patrick DL, Eagle J, and Hermalin JA: Collaboration, consultation and referral in an integrated health-mental program at an HMO. Social Work in Health Care *5*:833-896, 1979.

Coleman JV: "Interdisciplinary implications of health care," in Miller RS (Ed.): Primary Health Care: More Than Medicine. Englewood Cliffs (NJ), Prentice-Hall, 1983, pp. 113-120.

Collins J: Social Casework in General Medical Practice. London, Pitman, 1965.

Comley A: Family therapy and the family physician. Canadian Family Physician *19*:78-81, 1973.

Crane DD: The family therapist, the primary care physician, and the health maintenance organization: Pitfalls and possibilities. Family Systems Medicine *4*: 22-30, 1986.

Cummings NA: Prolonged (ideal) versus short term (realistic) psychotherapy. Professional Psychology, November:491-501, 1977.

Cummings WT and Follette WT: Psychiatric services and medical utilization in a prepaid health plan setting, Part II. Medical Care 6:31-41, 1968.

Dana B: "The Collaborative Process," in Miller RS and Rehr H (Eds.) Social Work Issues in Health Care. Englewood Cliffs (NJ), Prentice-Hall, 1983, pp. 181-220.

Dana B, Banta HD, and Deuschle KW: "An agenda for the future or interprofessionalism," in Rehr H (Ed.): Medicine and Social Work: An Exploration of Interprofessionalism. New York, Prodist, 1974.

Davis MM: Clinics, Hospitals and Health Centers. New York, Harper, 1927.

Dayringer R: Family therapy techniques for the family physician. Journal of Family Practice 6:303-307, 1978.

Dingle JH, Badger GF, and Jordan WS: Illness in the Home. Cleveland, Case Western Reserve University Press, 1964.

Doherty WJ: Family interventions in health care. Family Relations 34:129-137, 1985.

Doherty WJ and Baird MA: Family Therapy and Family Medicine. New York, Guilford Press, 1983.

Dongray M: Social work in general practice. British Medical Journal 2:1220-1223, 1958.

Dongray M: Co-operation in general practice: A medical social worker replies to a doctor. Almoner 14(12):547-556, 1962.

Dubos RJ: Mirage of Health. New York, Harper & Row, 1979.

Dym B: Personal communication, 1984.

Dym B: Collaborative work: The primary care health team. Working Together 1(3):9, 1986.

Dym B and Berman S: Family systems medicine: Family therapy's next frontier? Family Therapy Networker 9 (1):20, 1985.

Dym B and Berman S: The primary health care team: Family physician and family therapist in joint practice. Family Systems Medicine 4 (1):9-21, 1986.

Engel GL: The need for a new medical model: A challenge for biomedicine. Science 196:129-136, 1977.

Engel GL: The clinical application of the biopsychosocial model. American Journal of Psychiatry 137:535-544, 1980.

Engels F: The Condition of the Working Class in England. Moscow, Progress Publishers, 1973.

Epstein NB and Levin S: Training for family therapy within a faculty of medicine. Canadian Psychiatric Association Journal 18:203, 1973.

Epstein NB, Levin S, and Bishop DS: The family as a social unit. Canadian Family Physician 22:1411-1413, 1976.

Epstein NB, Bishop DS, and Levin S: The McMaster model of family functioning. Journal of Marriage and Family Counseling 4:19, 1978.

Estes R (Ed.): Health Care and the Social Services: Social Work Practice in Health Care. St. Louis, Warren H. Green, 1984.

Fleck S: Family functioning and family pathology. Psychiatric Annals *10*:46-57, 1980.

Follette WT and Cummings NA: Psychiatric services and medical utilization in a prepaid health plan setting. Medical Care *5*:25-35, 1967.

Forman JAS and Fairbairn EM: Social Casework in General Practice. London, Oxford University Press, 1968.

Freidson E: Profession of Medicine: A Study of the Sociology of Applied Knowledge. New York, Harper & Row, 1970.

Friedman M: Pathogenesis of Coronary Artery Disease. New York, McGraw-Hill, 1969.

Garner A and Weinar C: The Mother-Child Interaction in Psychosomatic Disorders. Urbana, University of Illinois Press, 1959.

Geiger HJ: "The meaning of community oriented primary care in the American context," in Connor and Mullen (Eds.): Community Oriented Primary Care: New Directions for Health Services Delivery. Washington, DC, National Academy Press, 1983, pp. 60-103.

Gilchrist IC, Gough JB, Horsfall-Turner YR et al: Social work in general practice. Journal of the Royal College of General Practice *28*:675-686, 1978.

Ginzberg E: The monetarization of health care. New England Journal of Medicine *310*:1161-1165, 1984.

Glenn ML: Family illness rituals. Journal of Family Practice *14*:950-954, 1982.

Glenn ML: On Diagnosis: A Systemic Approach. New York, Brunner/Mazel, 1984.

Glenn ML: Toward collaborative family-oriented health care. Family Systems Medicine *3*:466-475 (1985).

Glenn ML, Atkins L, and Singer RE: Integrating a family therapist into a family medical practice. Family Systems Medicine *2*:137-145, 1984.

Goldberg EM: Family Influences of Psychosomatic Illness. London, Tavistock, 1958.

Goldberg EM and Neill JE: Social Work in General Practice. London, George Allen and Unwin, 1972.

Greene GJ and Kruse KA: Social work in family practice: What are the prospects? Unpublished manuscript.

Greene GJ, Kruse KA, and Arthurs RJ: Family practice social work: A new area of specialization. Social Work in Health Care *10*(3):53-73, 1985.

Hall A and Fagan R: "Definition of a System," in Ruben BD and Kim JY (Eds.): General Systems Theory and Human Communication. Rochelle Park, Hayden, 1978.

The Health Units of Boston 1924-1933. City of Boston Printing Department, 1933.

Hippocrates: Writings, translated by Jones WHS. Vol. I. Cambridge (MA), Loeb Classical Library, 1972 (1923).

Hoffman L: Foundations of Family Therapy. New York, Basic Books, 1981.

Huntington J: Social Work and General Medical Practice: Collaboration or Conflict? London, George Allen and Unwin, 1981.

Huygen FJA: Family Medicine: The Medical Life History of Families. Nijmegen (The Netherlands), Dekker & Van de Vegt, 1978.

Huygen FJA and Smits AJA: Family therapy, family somatics, and family medicine. Family Systems Medicine *1*:23-32, 1983.

Illich I: Medical Nemesis: The expropriation of Health. New York, Pantheon, 1976.

Johnston M: The work of a clinical psychologist in primary care. Journal of the Royal College of General Practice *28*:661-668, 1978.

Justin RG and Shanks JL: Treating psychosocial problems in solo family practice. Family Practice Research Journal *2*:258-270, 1983.

Kanner L: Children as organs of parental hypochondriasis. Child Psychiatry, 616, 1948.

Kantor D and Lehr W: Inside the Family. San Francisco, Jossey-Bass, 1975.

Kellner R: Family Ill Health: An Investigation in General Practice. New York, Charles C. Thomas, 1963.

Kerson T (Ed.): Social Work in Health Settings. New York, Longman, 1982.

Klein R, Dean A, and Bogdanoff M: The impact of disease upon the spouse. Journal of Chronic Diseases *20*:241-252, 1968.

Kraus AS and Lilienfield AM: Some epidemiological aspects of the high mortality rate in the young widowed group. Journal of Chronic Diseases *10*:207-215, 1959.

Kreitman N: The patient's spouse. British Journal of Psychiatry *110*:159-167, 1964.

Laszlo E: The Systems View of the World. New York, Braziller, 1972.

Levenson D: Montefiore: The Hospital as a Social Instrument. New York, Farrar, Straus, 1984.

Levine M: Psychotherapy in Medical Practice. New York, Macmillan, 1942.

Lipowski SJ, Lipsitt DR, and Whybrow PC (Eds.) Psychosomatic Medicine. New York, Oxford University Press, 1977.

Locke SE: Stress, Adaptation and Immunity. General Hospital Psychiatry, *4*:49-56, 1982.

Lowe JI and Herranen M: Conflict in teamwork: Understanding roles and relationships. Social Work in Health Care *3*:323-330, 1978.

Lynch JJ; The Broken Heart: The Medical Consequences of Loneliness. New York, Basic Books, 1977.

Madison DL: "Opportunities and constraints for community oriented primary care," in Connor and Mullen (Eds.): Community Oriented Primary Care: New Directions for Health Services Delivery. Washington, DC, National Academy Press, 1983, pp. 119-137.

Marinker M: Comments. Michigan conference on "The family in family medicine." Ann Arbor, June 20, 1982.

McGoldrick M and Gerson R: Genograms in Family Assessment. New York, W.W. Norton, 1985.

Medalie JM: Family Medicine: Principles and Applications. Baltimore, Williams and Wilkins, 1978.

Medalie JM: Comments. Michigan conference on "The family in family medicine." Ann Arbor, June 18, 1982.

Medalie JM, Snyder M, Groen JJ, et al: Angina pectoris among 10,000 men: Five year incidence and univariate analysis. American Journal of Medicine *55*:583, 1973.

Mertens A: Institute of Social Medicine, Nijmegen University Nijmegen, The Netherlands. Unpublished manuscript.

Meyer RJ and Haggerty RJ: Streptococcal infections in families: Factors altering individual susceptibility. Pediatrics *29*:539-549, 1962.

Miller RS (Ed.): Primary Health Care: More Than Medicine. Englewood Cliffs (NJ), Prentice Hall, 1983.

Miller RS and Rehr H (Eds.): Social Work Issues in Health Care. Englewood Cliffs (NJ), Prentice-Hall, 1983.

Minuchin S, Rosman BL, and Baker L: Psychosomatic Families. Cambridge (MA), Harvard University Press, 1978.

Mizrahi T and Abramson J: Sources of strain between physicians and social workers: Implications for social workers in health care settings. Social Work in Health Care *10*:33-51, 1985.

Olson DH, Sprenkle DH, and Russell CS: Circumplex model of marital and family systems: I. Cohesion and adaptability dimensions, family types, and clinical applications. Family Process *18*:3-28, 1979.

Parkes CM: Bereavement: Studies of Grief in Adult Life. New York, International Universities Press, 1972.

Parsons T: The Social System. New York, Free Press, 1964 (1951).

Patterson JM: Book Review: Health and Ways of Living: The Alameda County study, by Berkman LF and Breslow L. Family Systems Medicine *3*(1):111-114, 1985.

Peachey R: Family patterns of stress. General Practitioner *27*:82-89, 1963.

Pearse IH and Crocker LH: The Peckham Experiment. London, Allen and Unwin, 1943.

Phillips W and Mauksch L: Interview (by Michael Glenn). Family Systems Medicine *3*:344-355, 1985.

Rakel RE: Textbook of Family Practice, 3rd Edition. Philadelphia, Saunders, 1983.

Ransom DC: On why it is useful, to say that "the family is a unit of care" in Family Medicine: Comment on Carmichael's essay. Family Systems Medicine *1*(1):17-22, 1983a.

Ransom DC: Random Notes: The family as patient—What does this mean? Family Systems Medicine *1*(2):99-103, 1983b.

Ransom DC: Random Notes: The family as patient—Part II. Family Systems Medicine *1*(3):110-113, 1983c.

Ransom DC: Random Notes: The changing family: Implications for family practice. Family Systems Medicine 2:451-458, 1984.

Ransom DC: Random Notes: The family health maintenance demonstration. Family Systems Medicine 3:371-376, 1985.

Ransom DC and Grace NT: "Family therapy," in Rosen GM, Geyman JP, and Layton RH (Eds.): Behavioral Science in Family Practice. New York, Appleton-Century-Crofts, 1979.

Rees WD and Lutkins GS: Mortality of bereavement. British Medical Journal 4: 13-20, 1967.

Reiss D and Oliveri ME: Family stress and community frame. Marriage and Family Review 6:61-84 (1983).

Report to the President from The President's Commission on Mental Health, Vol 1. Washington, DC, U.S. Government Printing Office, 1978.

Richardson HB: Patients Have Families. New York, Commonwealth Fund, 1948.

Rosenblatt RA, Cherkin DC, Schneeweiss R, et al: The structure and content of family practice: Current status and future trends. Journal of Family Practice 15:681, 1982.

Schmidt DD: The family as the unit of medical care. Journal of Family Practice 7:303-313, 1978.

Schmidt DD: When is it helpful to convene the family? Journal of Family Practice 16:967-973, 1983.

Scott R: Medicine in society. Journal of the Royal College of General Practitioners 9:3-16, 1965.

Seifert M: Interview (by Michael Glenn). Family Systems Medicine 3:221-232, 1985.

Shanks JL: Expanding treatment for the elderly: Counseling in a private medical practice. Personnel and Guidance Journal, May:553-555, 1983.

Silver G: Family Medical Care: A Design for Health Maintenance. Cambridge (MA), Ballinger, 1974.

Starr P: The Social Transformation of American Medicine. New York, Basic Books, 1983.

Stephens GG: The Intellectual Basis of Family Practice. Tucson, Winter, 1982.

Stoeckel JD and Candib LM: The neighborhood health center: Reform ideas of yesterday and today. New England Journal of Medicine 280:1385-1391, 1969.

Sullivan HS: The Interpersonal Theory of Psychiatry. New York, Norton, 1953.

Szasz TS: The Myth of Mental Illness. New York, Harper & Row, 1974.

Szasz TS and Hollander MH: A contribution to the philosophy of medicine. Archives of Internal Medicine 97:585-592, 1956.

Taylor RB (Ed.): Family Medicine: Principles and Practice, 2nd Edition. New York, Springer-Verlag, 1983.

Ulrich R: Interview (by Michael Glenn). Family Systems Medicine 3:88-102, 1985.

Virchow R: Disease, Life, and Man, translated by Rather LJ. Stanford, Stanford University Press, 1958.

Waitzkin H: The social origins of illness. International Journal of Health Services *11*:77-103, 1981.

Walsh F: Normal Family Processes. New York, Guilford Press, 1982.

Watzlawick, P, Beavin J, and Jackson JJ: Pragmatics of Human Communication. New York, W.W. Norton, 1967.

Weakland JH: "Family somatics": A neglected edge. Family Process *16*:263-272, 1977.

Wise H: The primary care health team. Archives of Internal Medicine *130*:438-444, 1972.

Wise H, Beckhard R, Rubin I, and Kyte AL: Making Health Teams Work. Cambridge (MA), Ballinger, 1974.

Worby C: Remarks, Michigan conference on "The family in Family Medicine." June 19, 1982.

Young M, Benjamin B, and Walks C: Mortality of widowers. Lancet *ii*:454, 1963.

INDEX

Alcoholism, 33, 141; Alcoholics Anonymous, 108; family history of, 47; social medicine and, 59

Almoner. (*see* Social workers)

Ambulatory care, prepaid plans and, 11

Angina: psychosocial factors in, 20; treatment of, 140

Anorexia, 53

Antonovsky, A., 31-32

Anxiety, 8; CHC model and, 111; childhood, 54; chronic, 189; coping with, 140

Asthma, treatment of, 140

Attendance patterns, 20

Auto-immune illnesses, 21

Baird, M., 111-112, 114, 141, 168, 182, 189-192

Bassoff, B.Z., 171

Behavior: of family, 18-21, 24-25; motivation for, 47; patterns, 44; recurrent, 24; systems approach to, 23

Bereavement: grief work, 99; illnesses and, 20; short-term therapy and, 76

Berkman, L., 29-30

Bernard, C., 59

Billing. (*see* Reimbursement)

Biomedical model, 85; dominance of, 4; in family medicine, 8, 98; insurance and, 5, 9-10; renaissance of, 11-12, 88

Biopsychosocial model: HMOs and, 12-14; history of, 4; psychosomatic disorders, 18-21, 140-141, 188;

[Biopsychosocial model] (*see also* Collaborative health care; Psychosocial disorders)

Candib, L.M., 61-62, 183-184

Cardiovascular disease, 20, 140

Carmichael, L., 90-91

Case management, conjoint, 118-122

Casework services, 69-77. (*see also* Social Work; Therapy)

Catchment area, 39

Causality, circular, 23-24

Chains, health care, 3, 11-12. (*see also* Health maintenance organizations)

Change: crisis points and, 187; stress from, 55; systems theory of, 23-24

Charts, in CHC, 195, 198

CHC. (*see* Collaborative health care)

Child care, 4

Christie-Seely, J., 29, 114, 188

Chronic pain syndrome, 140

Cigarette smoking, 33-34

City hospitals, 63

Clinics: in academic settings, 128-129; CHC model, 95; community-based, 42, 61-64, 86, 100; ethnic-based, 70; mental health, 199; public health, 125-126; rural, 86; satellite, 96-97, 127; tertiary, 98-99; voluntary principle, 61

Co-billing. (*see* Reimbursement)

Coherence, 31-32

Collaborative health care (CHC): basis for, 89-95; charts in, 195-196; collapse of, 88-89; collegial search

[Collaborative health care]
in, 130-133; communication in,
134-136; economic rationale for,
34; family-oriented, 95-101; history of, 57, 69-87; HMO, 125-127;
interprofessional conflict in, 160-
179; physician-therapist in, 116-
117; private practice models, 106-
124; in public settings, 124-125;
resistance to, 204; systems perspective in, 23; types of, 105-129
Communication: in CHC settings,
134-136; family patterns. (*see*
Family dynamics)
Communities: catchment area, 39;
CHC clinics, 100; community nursing, 94; defined, 35-43; ethnic,
39-40; interfacing, 37; minority,
83; outreach, 86; provider's view
of, 40; regnant, 42; social unit,
63
Community-based health care, 4, 13,
35; Civil Rights movement and,
86; clinics, 42, 61-64, 86, 100;
family-oriented, 95; economic
problems of, 166-167; history of,
57, 82-83; macrosystems approach,
87; movement, 82-87; nationwide
network of centers, 63; social
work in, 70, 77; team approach,
71, 96; therapy services, 125
Competition, among providers, 204.
(*see also* Profit motive)
Compliance, patient, 28, 110-111;
family dynamics of, 142-148;
referral for therapy and, 182
Confidentiality, in CHC, 196
Conjoint therapy, 110-115, 118-122
Consumers, community of, 41-42.
(*see also* Patients)
Contextual medicine, 17
Continuing education, 171

Coping: medical model, 32; of normal families, 81
Corporate medicine: chains, 3, 11-12;
costs and, 10-11, 162; profit motive of, 11, 14
Cost(s): cost-control rules, 5; cost-
effective care, 4, 85, 204; generalists and, 90; HMOs and, 100, 125,
165-166; malpractice and, 201;
primary care movement and, 92;
psychiatric disorders and, 162; reorganization and, 9-11
Counseling: conjoint, 110; continuum, 113; by family physicians,
51, 114-115, 167-168; in HMOs,
101; insurance and, 11; mistrust
of, 87; on-site, 110; physician-
therapist skills, 52; in primary
care, 29, 112; private practice,
174; therapy techniques, 113
(*see also* Family therapy; Therapy)
Counselors. (*see* Therapist/counselors)
Crane, D.D., 126
Crisis: mobile crisis care units, 86;
patient's family and, 47-48; referral and, 187; short-term therapy
and, 76 systems theory and, 23-
24
Crocker, L.H., 67

Davis, M., 61-62
Death, 20; of females, 30-31; grief
work, 9; of infants, 86; short-
term therapy and, 76; social networks and, 29-30
Depression reaction, 8, 54; CHC and,
111; chronic, 189; coping with,
140
Diagnosis: biomedical model and, 10;
codes, 5, 9; DSM-III, 126, 162;

[Diagnosis]
mutual, 109; reimbursement and, 11
Diet, 33. (*see also* Eating disorders)
Disability, social workers and, 70, 74
Disease. (*see* Illness)
Districts, health care, 39, 62
Doherty, W., 111-114, 141, 168, 182, 189-192
Drug abuse, 54, 111, 196, 198
Dubos, R.J., 58-60
Dym, B., 118-121

Eating disorders, 18, 53
Education: continuing, 171; of families, 77, 112; medical, 96, 128-129, 203; nurse educators, 108; of patient, 92, 109
Emergency care: centers, 14; chain facilities, 11
Emotional problems. (*see* Psychosocial disorders)
Engel, G., 92
Engels, F., 59-60
Estes, E., 77
Ethics, costs and, 10
Ethnic communities, 39-40, 83
Evaluation, in team care, 85

Fairbairn, A.M., 72
Family: adjunctive treatment of, 139; CHC model and, 95-101; convening criteria, 183; current trends in, 44-45; defined, 24, 43; disturbed, 189; health centers for, 64-68; health maintenance checkup of, 139; household as, 44; life cycle and, 65, 114; longitudinal studies of, 78; nuclear model of, 45; psychosomatic, 188; social develop-

[Family]
ment of, 67; as stressor, 20; subjective criteria for, 46-48; as unit of illness, 79 (*see also* Family dynamics; Family medicine; Family therapy)
Family dynamics, 4, 9; illness and, 16-34; interrelationships, 5; patient and, 49; patterns in, 47; somatic approach to, 18-21
Family Health Maintenance Demonstration project, 80-82
Family medicine, 91; biomedical model, 8, 98; brief therapy in, 28; conflict in, 167-168; controversy in, 91; development of, 89; family physicians, 89-91; family therapy in. (*see* Family therapy); history of, 6, 98; mainstreaming of, 90; patient constructs in, 49; relational model, 90-91; rise of, 87; social workers in, 77, 178; systems theory and, 111; trends in, 6; women in, 91, 173-174; working with families in, 29, 51, 114-115, 167-168
Family Systems Medicine, 17
Family systems theory, 111
Family therapy: continuum of, 111-112; in general medical practice, 28-29, 52; history of, 9-10; maturity of, 87, 89; motivation for, 183-193; and physical illness, 93; referral for, 183-193; "working with families" vs., 29, 51, 114-115, 167-168
Fats, dietary, 33
Fee(s): in CHC, 131; fee-for-service practice, 38, 163-165; therapist's, 116 (*see also* Costs)
Feedback. (*see* Communication)
For-profit organizations. (*see* Corporate medicine; Profit motive)

Forman, J.A.S., 72

Funding, 84-85, 201. (*see also* specific project)

Gatekeeper concept: CHC model and, 96; in HMOs, 126; primary care physician and, 13, 92; teams as, 13

Geiger, H., 37-38

General practitioners: as gatekeepers, 92; medical social workers and, 74; patient relationships with, 173-177; preference for, 90; therapy and, 87

Genogram, 44

Goldberg, E.M., 71-72, 75-76

Grace, N.T., 184

Great Society, 82

Greene, G., 77

Grief work, 9

Grose, N., 106-107, 155

Group medical practice

Group practice: CHC model, 95-101; community and, 41; private, 3; social workers in, 72-75 (*see also* Health maintenance organizations)

Health activists, 83

Health care system, 25-28; consumers of, 41-42; decentralized, 62; macrosystems, 87; movements, 61-64; self-service, 66; volunteers and, 61 (*see also* specific providers)

Health clinics. (*see* specific types)

Health coordinators, 108-110

Health demonstration projects, 63. (*see also* specific project)

Health educators. (*see* Education)

Health insurance. (*see* Insurance, health)

Health maintenance organizations (HMOs): access to care rules, 5;

[Health maintenance organizations] CHC model in, 96, 100-101, 125-128; closed-panel, 199; community and, 40; family practice-oriented, 12-14; history of, 80-82; incentives in, 165-166 profit motives of, 11, 125; reimbursement in, 122; satellite clinics, 127; size of, 11; specialist-based, 14

Health Insurance Plan (HIP) project, 80-82, 125

Health workers. (*see* Professionals)

Hippocrates, 57-59

HMOs. (*see* Health maintenance organizations)

Holistic health approach, 95; CHC and, 122-124; family medicine and, 90; HMOs and, 100 (*see also* Family medicine)

Home care, 75

Hospice care, 9

Hospitals, 11; medical social work in, 70; as organizing centers, 83; psychiatric, 198; tertiary-care, 77, 98-99

Households, 8, 43-45. (*see also* Family)

Huntington, J., 172, 174-175, 177

Huygen, F.J.A., 53, 186-187

Hypochondriasis, 8, 18

Illich, Ivan, 4

Illness: biopsychosocial model of, 91; chronic, 70; family as unit of, 79; generational development of, 25; iatrogenic, 4; occupational, 59-60; patterns of, 20; psychosocial context, 7-8, 16-18, 52-55, 60, 171, 185; somatic fixation, 8, 53, 146; stress-related, 8, 20; symptoms of, 25, 112, 144, 184, 188-189; terminal, 9, 76

Immune system, stress and, 20

Incest, 144
Infant mortality, 86
Infections, stress and, 20-21
Insurance, health, 171; access to therapy and, 162; biomedical model and, 9-10; co-billing, 121; codes of, 162; diagnostic nosology, 5; therapists and, 99 (*see also* Medicaid; Medicare)
Interdisciplinary programs. (*see* Team care)
Internal medicine, 82; primary care movement and, 92; on teams, 86
Irritable bowel syndrome, 8, 53-54

Job descriptions, 178

Kark, S., 80
Kellner, R., 19
Kinship, 43-46

Lead poisoning, 86, 166
Levine, M., 78
Licensing, 171
Life stress illness, 16
Living arrangements. (*see* Households)

McMaster model, 28, 113
Macy Foundation Study, 78-80
Malpractice, 5; costs of, 201; potential suits, 26, 176
Manahan, W., 122
Marital therapy, 9
Marriage, mortality and, 30 (*see also* Families)
Meals on Wheels, 75
Medicaid, 10, 82, 85, 162; reimbursement policies, 121, 164-165; therapists and, 99, 199; wellness programs and, 124

Medical Committee for Human Rights, 83
Medical model. (*see* Biomedical model)
Medical practice, 50-52. (*see also* by type)
Medical records, CHC, 195-196
Medical social work, 70, 99, 175
Medicare, 10, 82, 162; therapists and, 99
Mental health services: CHC and, 93; and community primary care, 83; cost of, 162; in HMO, 166; in primary care clinics, 87; social workers and, 70, 77 (*see also* Family therapy; Therapy)
Migraine, 54, 140, 189
Minuchin, S., 16, 19, 111
Montefiore program, 80-82. (*see* HIP)
Mortality. (*see* Death)
Myocardial infarction: psychosocial factors, 20; systems approach and, 28

National Health Services Act (1947), 72
National Social Unit Organization, 62-63
Neighborhood clinics, 42; as community, 40; health workers in, 62
Neill, J.E., 71-72, 75-76
Neurodermatitis, 8
Neurosis: illness and, 19; referrals and, 188
Nuclear family, 45
Nurses: educators, 108; nurse practitioners, 86, 88, 95; primary care and, 99; psychosocial approach by, 94; social work disputes with, 171; on teams, 86
Nursing homes, chains, 11, 14
Nutrition, 18, 33, 53

Obesity, 18
Obstetrics-gynecology, primary care
    movement and, 92
Occupational communities, 40-41
Occupational health, 33, 59-60
Ombudsmen, 77
Outreach programs, 86

PPOs. (*see* Private medicine practice)
Pastoral counseling, 9; defined, 48;
    diagnosis with, 109; education of,
    86
Patients: advocates for, 77, 83; af-
    fective ties of, 46-48; compliance
    of, 28, 110-111, 142-148, 182;
    confidentiality of, 197; conflicts
    with, 160; as consumers, 41-42;
    defined, 48; education programs,
    86, 124; emotional problems of,
    105; expectations of, 181; family
    system as, 24-25; hidden, 48; liv-
    ing arrangements of, 43-46; psy-
    chosocial needs of, 71, 120, 167;
    screening evaluations, 138; social
    networks of, 29-33; as staff, 86
Payment. (*see* Reimbursement)
Pearse, I.H., 67
Peckham Experiment, 64-68, 97
Pediatricians: primary care movement
    and, 92; team care and, 86
Peptic ulcer disease, 140
Phillips, C., 62-63
Physician: autonomy of, 5; as biol-
    ogists, 66-67; as consultants, 79;
    counseling skills of, 29, 51, 114-
    115, 167; dominant expertise of,
    50, 113, 173; as gatekeepers, 13,
    170; as generalists, 6; glut of, 87-
    88; legal jeopardy of, 176; patient
    conflicts, 184-185; patient rela-
    tionship, 175-176; as therapist,
    51-52; therapist referrals by, 115,
    167 (*see also* by practice type)

Physician assistants, 88, 98
Pioneer Health Centers, 64-68
Placebo effect, 51
Poverty: access to care and, 125, 201-
    202; get-tough policy, 88; reform
    programs, 82-87
Premise of significance, 18
Prepaid plans, 80; ambulatory care
    and, 11 (*see also* Health mainten-
    ance organizations)
President's Commission on Mental
    Health (1978), 7
Preventive care, 4; in CHC practice,
    138-139, 186; critical care vs., 11;
    evaluation of, 89; in families, 112,
    186; HMOs and, 100; history of,
    33-34; nonreimbursable, 5; profes-
    sionals and, 80; role of, 92-93
Primary care medicine, 6; CHC in,
    95-101, 138-159; community
    oriented, 38, 84-86; counseling
    skills and, 168; family-focused
    (*see* Family medicine); movement,
    91; specialties and, 91-93; team
    interdependence, 86; therapist in,
    118-122; training programs for,
    128
Private medical practice, 3, 13, 65;
    access to care in, 170; CHC in,
    99, 105-124; reimbursement is-
    sues, 14, 163-165; social workers
    in, 70-77 (*see also* by practice
    type)
Professionals: conflicts among, 99,
    135, 160-179, 200-201, 203; cul-
    tural differences, 172; fit between,
    106, 117, 131; health center move-
    ment and, 61-62; radical, 83, 87;
    role difficulty in, 26, 81-82, 169-
    170; sex-role differences, 173-175;
    therapy as, 51 (*see also* specific
    professions)
Profit motive, 3, 5; of chains, 11;
    of HMOs, 100, 125, 165-166;

[Profit motive]
insurance coverage a.1d, 10; values and, 171
Providers. (*see* Professionals)
Psychiatry: biochemical diseases and, 5, 80; consultation-liaison in, 19, 87, 99 (*see also* Mental health services)
Psychosocial disorders, 16-18; frequency of, 7-8; physician attitudes and, 182; politics of, 171; referrals for, 185
Psychosomatic disorders: family somatic approach, 18-21, 28-29, 52, 111, 188; referral for, 185; treatment of, 140-141
Psychotherapy. (*see* Family therapy; Therapy)
Public health programs, 59; CHC in, 124-125; history of, 61-64; nurses in, 94; social workers and, 69-77

Ransom, D.C., 44-45, 49, 82, 184
Red Cross, 63
Referrals, 87; in CHC, 131; from family practice, 115-116; to family therapy, 106-107, 182; premature, 190; problems in, 180-194; self, 173; social workers and, 74-76; triangulation in, 192
Reimbursement: CHC and, 121, 132, 162; codes, 5; competititon for, 171; eligibility for, 164; fee-for-service, 14, 163-165; laws governing, 162; of social workers, 174; of therapists, 99, 121-122; types of, 10
Reiss, D., 37, 42
Richardson, H.B., 19, 71, 78-80
Robert Wood Johnson Foundation, 84
Role, professional strains, 26, 81-82, 169-170 CR Professionals

Rules, access to care, 5
Rural health clinics, 86

Salutogenesis, 31
Schizophrenics, 18-19, 54
Schmidt, D.D., 17-18, 183
Scott, R., 72
Seifert, M., 108-110
Self-help, 83, 86, 95, 173
Sexual abuse, 144
Short-term therapy, 76
Sickle cell disease, 86
Silver, G.A., 80-82
Singer, R., 116
Single parents, 45
SOAP form, 196
Social medicine, 59-63
Social networks, 17, 29-33, 37
Social problems. (*see* Psychosocial disorders)
Social service agencies, 73-74
Social workers: biopsychosocial model, 175; CHC model and, 69-77; cultures of, 172; family therapy-oriented, 94, 178; medical, 70, 99, 175; mistrust of, 83; in private practice, 171, 176; reimbursement for, 201; role strains of, 169-179; on teams, 86
Socialized medical care, CHC in, 97
Somatic fixation, 8, 53, 146
Somatic symptoms, 144, 188
Specialists, medical, 6, 11; fragmentation and, 199; primary care services and, 92
Spiritual groups, 40
Stress: acute situational, 8; chronic strain, 20; psychosomatic premise and, 5, 18, 140-141; subjectivity of, 31; therapy and, 55-56, 76
Substance abuse, 9, 54, 111; confidentiality and, 196; hospitalization for, 198; treatment of, 141

Symptoms, somatic, 8, 53, 112, 144, 146, 188; generational development of, 25; unexplained, 184, 189

Systems theory, 21-28, 93; family and, 24-25, 111; *milieu interieur*, 59

Szasz, T., 4

Teaching programs, medical, 112, 173, 203; faculty in, 128-129; team approach, 96

Team care, 13; biomedical model, 86; costs and, 84-85, 88; decision-making on, 134-136; nurses and, 94; patient-physician and, 75; politics and, 86; professional conflicts in, 81-82, 88, 160-179; social workers and, 69-77 (*see also* Collaborative health care)

Tension headaches, 54, 140, 189

Terminal illness, 9, 76

Tertiary care, 77, 98-99

Therapist/counselors, 118-122, 181; gender of, 193; in group practice, 73; marketplace and, 171; in private practice, 174; referral to, 181-194

Therapy, 7, 78, 165; billing for, 121, 162; conjoint, 110-115, 118-122; continuum of, 113; counseling vs., 113-114; covert, 55; defined, 50-51; family (*see* Family therapy); HMOs and, 100-101; in general practice, 78; in group practices,

[Therapy] 73; short-term, 76; skills levels in, 190

Third-party payments. (*see* Insurance, health; Reimbursement)

Training: CHC and, 87; of physicians, 96, 128-129, 112, 173, 203; of primary care therapist, 119; team approach and, 96

Type A personality, 20

Ulrich, R., 84-86

Union health programs, 63

Valentine Lane Family Practice, 84-86

Values: assumptions and, 35; costs and, 10

Visiting nurses, 94

Wellness care. (*see* Holistic health approach)

Women: health movement of, 83, 86, 95; in medicine, 91, 173-174; mortality rates of, 30-31; referrals and, 75

Women and Infant Care program, 4

Working with the family concept, 29, 51, 114-115, 167-168; family therapy referral and, 188

YMCA, 66

ABOUT THE AUTHOR

Michael L. Glenn, M.D. is a family physician in Everett, Massachusetts. He works in a setting with two other family physicians and three family therapists. Dr. Glenn was one of the founders of the journal *Family Systems Medicine*, and serves as its book review editor and associate editor. He holds a faculty position at the University of Massachusetts Medical School in Worcester, Massachusetts.